KETO DIET FOR WOMEN OVER 50

SIMPLE GUIDE AND COOKBOOK SPECIFICALLY FOR WOMEN OVER 50 WHO WANT TO FOLLOW THE KETOGENIC DIET, TO LOSE WEIGHT AND IMPROVE HEALTH

By

Gianni SALVADORI

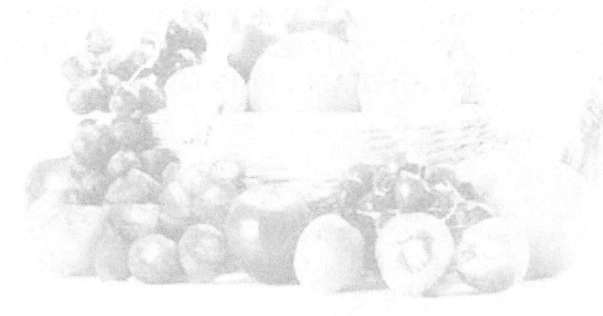

TABLE OF CONTENS

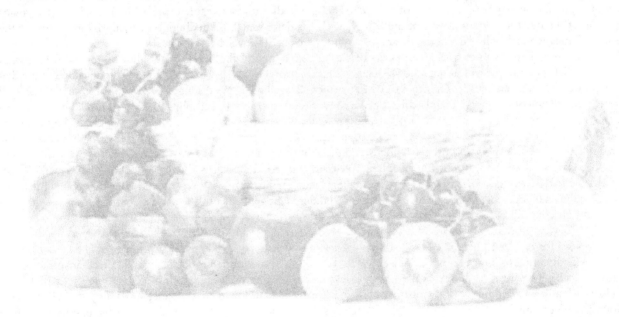

INTRODUCTION

The ketogenic diet is a diet based on the ability of our organism to use the lipid reserves when the availability of carbohydrates undergoes a significant reduction. The reserves available to the human body are many: the reserve represented by adipose tissue, which in an average individual is equal to 70 kg, is an unlimited source of energy while the one consisting exclusively of carbohydrates reaches total exhaustion in a short time. The ketogenic diet what it is about legend What to avoid and what to take? Cyclic ketogenic diet Physical activity Epilepsy Pregnancy Hashimoto's Thyroid Supplements Tissues receive energy in proportion to the actual availability of substrates in the blood: if lucose is present within acceptable levels is used by tissues that get energy on the contrary if the concentrations are insufficient then here are activated the following mechanisms: - glycogenolysis that converts fatty acids into energy - gluconeogenesis that transforms amino acids such as alanine and glutamine into sugars. The process of degradation of fat storage leads to the formation of ketone bodies (acetone, acetoacetate and beta-hydroxybutyric acid) by the liver, which in conditions of fasting and severe reduction of carbohydrates will be responsible for the onset of ketosis. This ketosis occurs physiologically in the morning after overnight fasting or following intense physical performance and can indicate a problem when the concentration of ketone bodies in the blood goes from 0.1 mmol/l up to about 7-8 mmol/l. The excess ketones, not used in the tissues, will be eliminated by respiration in the form of acetone that will determine the acetoxic breath and through the urine, where instead the excess of acidity is buffered by the simultaneous elimination of sodium, potassium and magnesium. Ketosis determines changes in the concentration of various hormones and nutrients, including ghrelin, amylin and leptin and, of course, of ketone bodies themselves. It is probably through these changes that one of the most important effects of the ketogenic diet is determined: the reduction or total disappearance of the feeling of hunger which will lead to a significant loss of body weight. The weight loss expected by following the ketogenic diet ranges from 1 to 2 kg per week, with peaks of 2.5 kg depending on the body weight and the regime followed. A ketogenic diet is composed as follows: - 70-75% fats - 20-25% proteins - 5-10% carbohydrates The objective of the diet is to induce and maintain ketosis. The types of dietary protocols used so far are distinguished by the amounts of the lipid and carbohydrate component. - Standard Ketogenic Diet (SKD): diet low in carbohydrates (5%), moderate in protein (20%) and high in fat (75% saturated fat). Fat and protein will be defined according to the weight of the person in question and the calories taken daily; - Cyclic ketogenic diet (CKD): consisting of a first phase with adherence to the ketogenic diet (5 days) and a second phase focused on carbohydrate intake (2 days). - Targeted ketogenic diet (TKD): diet that allows you to take carbohydrates when you train. Preferred are easily digestible carbohydrates with a high glycemic index. After workouts are over, protein intake is increased for muscle recovery and after that you continue to consume fat. - High protein ketogenic diet: similar to a standard ketogenic diet but with a higher protein intake the ratio of macronutrients will be: 60% fat, 35% protein and 5% carbohydrates. The ketogenic diet is strongly recommended in cases of: - Severe Obesity; - Diabetes Mellitus type 2; - Hepatic steatosis or "fatty liver"; - Polycystic ovary syndrome; - Acne; - Need for rapid slimming in case of pathologies related to excess eating - Pre-bariatric surgery The ketogenic diet is strongly discouraged in case of: - Subjects with BMI < 25 and nutrient deficiencies - Renal insufficiency; - Cardiovascular diseases Signs and symptoms that could be manifested by leading a diet of this type are: - Metabolic acidosis - Nausea and vomiting - Constipation - Glucose profile alterations - Kidney stones - Heart rhythm alterations - Gout. In order to minimize these effects it is advisable to start with a diet low in carbohydrates for the first weeks before eliminating them completely. A ketogenic diet can also modify the water and salt balance of the body, therefore it may be helpful to take a mineral supplement and a greater daily hydration to promote the elimination of ketone bodies. During the treatment with this diet may persist alterations of the alvo, more frequently constipation, and manifest alterations of blood chemistry parameters.

AUTHOR'S NOTE: This book has given you all the information you need to do this diet correctly and do it right. It is essential to understand what you are getting into when you embark on this diet, and this book gave you valuable information that you can use to your advantage and avoid the problems that can come with this diet. You want to stay healthy and make sure that your body can do what it needs to do. As with anything, we emphasize that if something seems wrong or unnatural, you will need to see a doctor to make sure you are safe and that your body can handle this diet. Use the knowledge in this book to get amazing recipes and learn directions for excellent meals for yourself. Consult your doctor before to starting new diet.

INTRODUCTION by Mynutritional di Susanna Agnello, Via del Ghironcello n.1 - 55100 Lucca P.Iva 06319310485 and with the realization of Sempoint di Fabio CIONI

TIPS FOR THE DIET

WHAT YOU SHOULD EAT

Like fasting, ketogenic thinning prompts you to eat.

On a keto diet, you should simply eat low-carb, attractive in protein, and high-fat foods.

MEAT

Eat only meats that are ideal in protein and low in carbohydrates, such as ground sirloin, tip, etc.

VEGETABLEs

Eat so-called "green" vegetables like turnips, kale, spinach, and kale. You can also eat ground vegetables, such as broccoli, squash, cauliflower, and zucchini. High-fat dairy products High-fat sustenance is somewhat standard on a ketogenic diet. Fat makes you feel full for a longer period. Delineations: high-fat cream, margarine and unusual cheeses.

NUTS AND SEEDS

Nuts and seeds are squeezed together with specific substances that help keep the body slim and healthy. Examples are macadamia, almonds, walnuts and sunflower seeds.

BERRIES AND SWEETENERS

Use sweeteners that have negligible sugar content, such as Splenda, Stevia, etc.

DISTINCTIVE FATS

Other sources of fat you can include in the keto diet are the high-fat portions related to the dressing of mixed vegetables, coconut oil, and soaked fats. Keep in mind that a typical ketone diet typically follows a plan with 70 percent fat, 25 percent protein, and 5 percent carbohydrate. It is recommended to consistently acquire between 20-30g of net carbs to consume fewer calories. Regardless, if the goal is to hit ketosis quickly, then reducing carbs and maintaining low glucose levels may be considered. While getting fitter is one of the goals of the keto diet, controlling total sugars and net starches is highly recommended. However, the urge to eat that occurs during the Keto diet can be alleviated by eating nuts, nut cream, cheddar cheese, and seeds.

BROCCOLI

Broccoli is an amazing food to eat regularly on a ketone diet as it is also rich in vitamins C and K. It is very important to consider that one serving of broccoli contains only 4g of net carbs. Empirical data and scientific examinations have shown that people who have type 2 diabetes can benefit from consuming broccoli, as this food reduces insulin resistance. Broccoli is considered a staple on a ketogenic diet.

ASPARAGUS

Asparagus is rich in vitamins C, A and K. It can help reduce tension and maintain a correct personality.

MUSHROOMS

Mushrooms have exceptional properties for balancing metabolic problems and therefore are essential in the Keto Diet.

THE PUMPKIN

Many types of squash are high in sugar. It is necessary to acquire only low-sugar types of pumpkins to keep the diet balanced. The best and most used is mid-year squash. Summer squash is occasionally used as a pasta substitute.

SPINACH

Spinach contains vitamins and minerals. In addition, it is a suitable food for heart health and reduces eye pain.

AVOCADO

It is high in fat, which makes it one of the best foods to be a fat supplement. It is rich in vitamin C and potassium.

GREEN BEANS

United in the vegetable family, green beans have fewer carbohydrates than various conventional products. One serving of green beans contains only 6g of net carbs, making it an important complement to any meal.

CAULIFLOWER

Known as the star of dishes, cauliflower is a versatile food that can be added to different types of meals.

It can be used for pizzas, wraps, dinners and mashed potatoes. With only 2 g of net sugars per serving, cauliflower is one of the main elements present and most used in low starch diets.

KALE AND LETTUCE

Used in servings of mixed greens, cabbage and lettuce are low-sugar items. They are an excellent source of vitamins A and C and help reduce threats of heart infections. In addition to being more nutritious than lettuce, kale also has more carbohydrates per serving. Consequently, it is necessary to pay attention to the quantity of black cabbage that is acquired in relation to the sugars contained in it and that the body igloba quickly.

WHAT NOT TO EAT

DON'T EAT GRAINS

Avoid eating grains such as rice, wheat and oats

SUGARS

Your sugar acquisition should be kept to a minimum

Avoid eating sweets, nectar, maple syrup.

TUBERS

If possible, avoid eating sweet potatoes, potatoes, etc. Furthermore, pay attention to the correct and controlled use of foods such as bananas, apples, melons, etc.

DANGERS AND SIDE EFFECTS OF THE KETOGENIC DIET AND HOW TO AVOID THEM

KETO FLU

Ethone dieters who switch to a fat-burning mode may experience early side effects, such as nausea, headache, cramps, mood swings, etc. Here are some things that can be done to alleviate the problem of these symptoms:

Gradual reduction of carbohydrates - You can prepare yourself for a ketonic diet by gradually reducing your carbohydrate intake. A sudden drop in carbohydrate intake can surprise your system, which can make you feel less well. A body that is not used to a low-carb diet takes some time to adjust. The sudden removal or drastic reduction of carbohydrates will fuel the brain with a weaker energy supply. Once the body has adapted to the diet and been fueled by ketones, these side effects disappear. A cup or two of broth a day should minimize the side effects of a ketone diet.

BAD BREATH

Dieters who follow a ketone diet or a low-carb diet can suffer from bad breath. This is caused by acetone, which is a ketone body. The aroma is usually described as a nail polish remover. Bad breath means that the body is turning into a fat burning machine and creating ketones to power the whole person and the brain. This smell can also be a body odor that usually occurs when you exercise or sweat a lot. It is worth noting that some people do not experience these symptoms. Other people have these symptoms only temporarily and then disappear over time once the body has adapted to the diet.

OTHER THINGS TO CONSIDER:

1. DRINK MORE WATER

It is normal to have a dry mouth when starting a low-carb diet for the first time. It is an indication that you have entered ketosis. It happens that you have less saliva in your mouth to brush your teeth and this can lead to bad breath It is therefore necessary to drink enough fluids and keep the body hydrated at all times. Salt is also a great oral cleansing ingredient.

2. ORAL HYGIENE

Maintaining good oral health is essential, especially when following a keto diet. Brushing your teeth more often doesn't always get rid of bad breath odor, but it can help minimize it and prevent it from mixing with other unpleasant odors.

3. REFRESHING FOR THE BREATH

A breath deodorant can be applied immediately and can somewhat mask the ketone odor present in your breath.

4. GIVE MORE TIME

In most cases, bad breath is only temporary, so it takes your body some time to get used to the diet to eliminate it.

If it doesn't go away after a few weeks or a month, a great way to deal with it is to reduce the level of ketosis. This can be done by eating more carbohydrates. Usually, people can get out of ketosis by adding 50-70g of carbohydrates, so the diet needs to be recalibrated. It is possible to alternate the intake of carbohydrates with intermittent fasting.

LEG CRAMPS

Leg cramps are common when starting a keto diet. Although leg cramps usually aren't a big deal, they can become so when they're painful. Leg cramps are caused by loss of magnesium due to increased urination. Here are three effective ways to prevent or treat leg cramps.

SALT AND WATER

The magical seawater blend can be reused to treat and prevent leg cramps. Always be well hydrated and drink enough fluids; this helps to curb the loss of magnesium.

MAGNESIUM SUPPLEMENT

Since leg cramps are caused by the reduction of magnesium, one way to treat them is to take magnesium in sachets or tablets. Alternatively, as a last resort, you can acquire more carbohydrates, which can weaken the effects of the ketone diet.

HIGH CHOLESTEROL LEVEL

A high-fat diet can cause side effects. Although a low-carb, high-fat diet like the Keto diet is known to improve the cholesterol profile, some people may experience some troubling results. It happens when the amount of good cholesterol exceeds the average level. Some tips to avoid these cases can be:

1 Reduction in the acquisition of fats

Since excessive fat consumption is the cause of the cholesterol increase, it is necessary to reduce the acquisition of fat, especially when you are not hungry. Also, choose low-fat drinks.

2 Intermittent fasting

Intermittent fasting is a true fast but for a short time. This is a great way to lower your cholesterol level. For example, you can eat less for breakfast or even skip it. This remedy doesn't have to be done every day but only occasionally.

ALCOHOLIC DRINKS AND INTOXICATION

Following a ketonic or low-carb diet could also lead to intoxication as a side effect. Ingest alcoholic substances. This is because the liver is much more involved in the generation of ketones during the diet and can reduce their functioning in the digestion of alcoholic substances such as liqueurs. When starting a ketone diet it is necessary to decrease the ingestion of alcoholic substances and liqueurs as the body has a lower tolerance to alcohol. This allows for regular maintenance of the program and an always healthy body. It must be said that sometimes carbohydrates can also release alcoholic substances So in addition to alcoholic beverages, you must also pay attention to the carbohydrates that contain them. If you decide to drink alcohol, among them, the Bloody Mary is a great choice with only 7g of carbohydrates, while a glass of margarita has 8g of carbohydrates and Cosmopolitan has 13g of carbohydrates. Not all drinks are prepared the same, so check the carbohydrates they contain (usually written on the bottle or can). Champagne is also an excellent choice with only 1g of carbs per serving.

KETO RASH

Wear comfortable, weatherproof clothing. Wearing thick clothing is recommended for sweating.

Use air conditioning or an electric fan to keep from sweating. Keto Rash occurs when ketones are released as you sweat as the sweat dries on the skin. You can choose to participate in less intense exercise programs that lead to lower levels of sweating. If the goal is just to lose weight, walking and exercising lightly are the right options

GIVE IT MORE TIME

If the diet program fails, the best way is to consult your doctor or simply get out of the state of ketosis. To get out of ketosis safely, you need to gradually add more carbohydrates to your diet. If the desire is still to lose weight, it is usually sufficient to add about 50-100g of carbohydrates to get out of ketosis and at the same time control the level of body weight. However, in this case the weight loss will be slower than when the body is in a state of ketosis.

Although the ketone diet can be used for the long term, it can also be followed for a short time. Getting out of ketosis is easy - gradually add carbohydrates to your diet. There are people who have had problems with Keto Rash the first time they went into ketosis. But it has been shown that from the second time you enter chest, it becomes less of a problem. Other times, Keto Rash doesn't even appear the second time you go into ketosis. So, if a person is seriously determined to follow a ketogenic diet, the advice is not to give up if "Keto Rush" occurs, but to try again and exploit this food system.

DRAWBACKS

As mentioned above, the ketogenic diet can have drawbacks, such as:

1. Low Energy Levels: People who have jobs that require high energy levels or athletes may find it difficult to start the ketogenic diet due to the reduced energy levels provided by the meal plan.

2. Restrictive Eating: There are rules to follow and you can't eat all you want.

3. Metabolic Issues: Critics also believe that following a low-carb diet for an extended period can disrupt healthy metabolic function Some people also tend to overdo a low-carb meal plan

EFFECTS OF THE KETOGENIC DIET

How the body uses various fuels. In the human body there are three primary "deposits" of fuel accumulation to which the body draws in case of need for a greater energy intake due to caloric deficiency. The body draws on its protein reserves to turn them into glucose in the liver. The body can tap into its carbohydrate reserve (glycogen). The body can also use its accumulation of fat, which is stored in the body as body fat.

There is also a fourth type of fuel the body can use, known as ketones. In an average diet, ketones are insignificant to the body for energy production. However, in a low-carb diet like the ketogenic diet, ketones are used a lot as a source of energy, especially by the brain. The tissues of the body always use the most available fuel source in the bloodstream. For example, if there is a high concentration of glucose in the body, the body chooses glucose as its preferred fuel source, except for organs such as the heart which use a mixture of glucose, ketones, and free fatty acids as fuel. If, however, there is a reduction in the concentration of glucose in the body, the body will have to choose the next available fuel source as an energy source. With a ketogenic diet, the body switches from using glucose as the primary source to using stored fat due to the increased availability of fat in the body. One of the goals of a ketogenic diet, therefore, is to increase the concentration of proteins and fats in the body relative to carbohydrates so that the accumulated excess fats are consumed to turn them into energy and thus eliminate the excess fat. There are other factors in the body besides reserves that help determine which fuels the body will use to get more energy. These include the levels of insulin, the glucagon hormones in the body, and the levels of regulatory enzymes to break down glucose and fat. The process by which these ketones are formed is what is known as ketogenesis and to understand the ketogenic diet it is essential to understand the concept of ketogenesis. Ketogenesis in the body depends on two main factors: the liver and fat cells. As blood insulin levels decrease, the mobilization of free fatty acids improves. It travels through the bloodstream aided by a protein known as albumin and, when in the blood, it can be used for energy production. Free fatty acids that are not used as fuel will be oxidized in the liver. This oxidation leads to the production of ketone bodies, which are then released into the bloodstream. Along with fat cells, the liver is another factor that determines ketogenesis in the body. The liver always produces ketones, with or without a ketogenic diet, but in small and insignificant quantities. The ketogenic diet, on the other hand, increases the amount of ketones present in the body. Therefore, when it is said that ketones are harmful by-products, it must be remembered that ketones are always present in the body and therefore indispensable. The liver is very essential for ketogenesis because, even though there are high levels of free fatty acids in the body, there would be no ketone production if the liver were not in a ketogenic state. The main function of liver glycogen is to help maintain healthy glucose levels. When following a low-carb diet and lowering blood glucose levels, liver glycogen prompts the liver to break down its glycogen stores in addition to releasing glucose into the bloodstream. The body uses this glucose for some time (between 12 and 16 hours depending on physical activity levels), after which time its glycogen stores are depleted. After exhaustion, ketogenesis increases rapidly based on the availability of free fatty acids. Metabolic effects of the ketogenic diet One thing critics are always quick to say when it comes to the ketogenic diet is that "the ketogenic diet will ruin your metabolism".

SO, WILL THE KETOGENIC DIET RUIN YOUR METABOLISM?

Your metabolic system is primarily aimed at making fuels available to your body whenever they are needed. As we continue to consume foods, the metabolic system continues to work to ensure that the energy from the foods is properly allocated and thus the excesses are stored. The average human being today, statistically, eats too much as a result, the metabolic system has more difficulty managing the work to be done than it should do as it was designed. During the hunger-generating diet, the metabolic system focuses on supplying glucose to the tissues that need it to make them function, such as the brain, kidneys, red blood cells, etc. This glucose is usually obtained from the body's protein stores; mainly muscle and sometimes fat. The metabolic system cannot determine how long this hunger state will last, whether a few hours or a few weeks It first tries to cope with the situation by acquiring the blood glucose supply and then detects some proteins from the muscles. But since it also needs to ensure that muscle mass is not excessively depleted, the body turns to ketones as a solution. Ketones can replace glucose and protein, so your muscles are spared from exhaustion and your body is balanced and fit thanks to the use of ketones as energy. This is what happens with a diet that generates hunger. On the other hand, on a low-carb diet, by eating some proteins and fats, muscles are unlikely to be depleted, as the proteins that are consumed are converted into glucose.

THERMAL EFFECT OF FOOD:
This energy breaks down the macronutrients from the foods consumed and processes them. Proteins use the highest amount of energy to distribute themselves. This is why low-carb diets improve metabolism. The same thing would also happen with any food that increases protein consumption and therefore not just the ketogenic diet.

THERMAL EFFECT OF THE ACTIVITY:
It refers to any form of activity that is not an indispensable bodily function. People who are physically inactive and live sedentary lifestyles can only burn 10-30% more calories than their BMR, but physically active people who exercise regularly consume more. So it's not just what we eat that affects metabolism. As long as you maintain a moderate level of physical activity and avoid complete hunger, you will be able to support a healthy metabolism.

WHAT NOT TO EXPECT FROM THE KETOGENIC DIET
Diet is not a miracle solution for weight loss. It is a lifestyle change that requires a lot of discipline and hard work to make it happen. However, once you get used to the diet rules, moments of pleasure and rapid weight loss begin. We cannot ignore the fact that the diet works without exercise. For best results, the ketogenic diet should be combined with regular exercise.

PRACTICAL ELEMENTS TO KEEP IN MIND

HOW DO I KNOW I AM IN KETOSIS?
There are some signs and symptoms like bad breath problems, increased thirst and dry mouth, increased urination and rapid weight loss is the sign that your body is in a state of ketosis.

HOW SHOULD I MONITOR MY KETONE LEVEL?
There are two methods of monitoring ketones, the first is urine test strips called keto strips. This is an inexpensive way to monitor ketone levels. Another method is blood testing, one of the most accurate methods for monitoring ketone levels. This method is expensive, you need a ketometer and strips to monitor your blood ketone level.

HOW DOES KETOSIS WORK IN MY BODY?
When we consume low-carb foods, our body uses fat as its primary energy source. Ketosis is the state where the breakdown of the liver into molecules is known as ketones. These ketones are used by our body for energy. In this state, your body breaks down fat for energy.

KETO DIET FOR WOMEN OVER 50

With the advancement of age, the body makes many changes some of which are beyond our control, such as genetic ones. Those related to daily life are instead more controllable. Therefore, the lifestyle that is maintained is very important for the balance of health. In the body of a woman many changes occur after 50 years and we can list them below

MENOPAUSE
The most significant change is menopause and there is no denying it. Menopause can drastically change a woman's body. Menopause does not actually pause anything, but it does change a woman's hormonal balance. Therefore, a woman's body, with menopause, must learn to find a new kind of balance due to hormonal change. Important are the symptoms that precede menopause such as night sweats, hot flashes and drastic mood swings. Sometimes there can be sleep disturbances and some women even go into depression. On the other hand, typical problems that are encountered after a woman experiences menopause can be urinary incontinence, known as pelvic prolapse. For those who have had children or are in a state of obesity, incontinence may occur more easily. In addition, weight gain can lead to the formation of fibroids in the uterus with the risk that these may enlarge over time and or turn into cancerous masses. Some of the symptoms of fibroids in the uterus are pelvic fullness, frequent urination, painful intercourse and heavy bleeding.

REDUCED BONE DENSITY
Several studies have shown that osteoporosis is a problem present more frequently in women than in men. It is a condition in which your bone becomes less dense, making your bones weak and thin. Therefore, they tend to break very easily. It is likely that one in, over fifty, women may experience a reduction in bone density. After the minus break, it is estimated that 30% of bone mass in a woman is literally lost. Worse is the case of a woman who experiences an early menopause, since the loss of bone density will be greater already when she will have reached the age of 55 years.

Therefore, when the woman is close to menonopause, a bone density examination is advisable. It is also necessary to have the doctor check the medications that are taken to avoid those that can induce a reduction in bone density loss.

MUSCLE LOSS

After the age of 50, there is a gradual decrease in muscle mass. This occurs not only in men but also in women. A decrease in physical strength also occurs. The best way to avoid this is to engage in strength training exercises such as squats or lunges two to three times a week. This will minimize the effects of strength loss. Or you can practice squats and lunges two to three times a week at home. Another benefit is regaining a better sense of balance.

WEAKER JOINTS

As you age, your joints will begin to become more fragile. This is not due to a reduction in bone density, but because the cartilage around the joints begins to wear away. These effects are felt more around 50 with the development of arthritis and joint pain; posture is also affected. It is necessary to avoid bending so that the body is not stressed and the joints are weakened. It is important to keep body weight under control. If the weight increases, it is necessary to take action to bring it back to the right value to avoid weakening the joints.

SIGNS OF AGING ON THE SKIN

With the passage of time on the skin can occur the appearance of spots and fine lines, as well as signs of sagging. These are indicators of aging. YesAlthough you maintain your skin very well and treat it daily, some signs of aging cannot be avoided. These signs will be worse especially if you did not take care of your skin during your youth, such as not using sunscreen while tanning. Also for some women during menopause it occurs that their skin becomes very dry and in need of moisturizing. The best way to deal with all these changes is to undergo regular health checkups to be aware of what is happening in your body.

MENOPAUSE AND KETO DIET

A woman with a diet plan that includes a higher carbohydrate intake may begin to see the signs generated by menopause earlier. How exactly can the ketogenic diet help you avoid the negative signs and effects of menopause?

CONTROL OF INSULIN LEVELS

For example, women adopting a ketogenic diet who suffer from polycystic ovary syndrome (PCOS) can help prevent their hormonal imbalance. Research studying low-glycemic diets has shown this relationship. PCOS causes an increase in insulin. So a low glycemic index carbohydrate diet could help ka insulin reduction and bring benefits.

LOSS OF FAT

Menopause can trigger metabolic treatment to alter and reduce fat. A recurring complaint in menopausal women is increased body weight and belly. A reduced level of estrogen commonly causes weight gain. A virtually carbohydrate-free diet is helpful in decreasing the muscle-to-fat ratio. Ketosis reduces hunger by controlling the development of the hormonal agent and food craving called ghrelin. During ketosis, the desire to eat is greatly reduced.

A DECREASE IN HOT FLASHES

No one widely understands hot flashes and why they occur, but it is certain that these derive from the hormonal variation from which these variations in body heat can arise.

Moreover it must be added regarding the ketogenic diet that the ketones that come constitute a solid source of energy for the mind. From reliable studies it has been demonstrated that ketones support the nerve centers therefore also the internal body temperature will be managed and regulated in a better way.

EXCELLENT NIGHT REST

Sleep will be better during a ketogenic diet due to a high intake of constant amounts of sugar. With the fact that hormones will undergo more substantial changes hot flashes will be less frequent, the pressure will be reduced and the body will relax better resulting in a better rest.

BENEFITS OF THE KETO DIET FOR WOMEN OVER 50 YEARS OLD

The keto diet has become popular because it is a very effective way to lose weight. But research also shows that not only does it help you lose weight, but it also brings great benefits to your health. When you use fat as fuel, your body becomes very active and stronger. The extra energy will help you do workouts and improve your endurance.

THE BENEFITS THAT WOMEN CAN GET FROM THE KETO DIET ARE:

INCREASED ENERGY LEVEL
Women over 50 don't have the same energy level as women in their 30s. They struggle to do workouts, but the Keyo diet helps increase your energy level and reduce weakness. When your energy level increases, your mind also functions better by focusing properly on the tasks at hand.

REDUCES ANXIETY AND DEPRESSION
The keto diet also helps in reducing anxiety. This is due to its high fat intake and low sugar level. A recent study also randomly showed that women who followed a Keto diet reduced their state of anxiety and depression as opposed to those who did not follow it.

PROTECTION AGAINST TYPE 2 DIABETES
The keto diet reduces sugar intake to less than 20 grams and helps type 2 diabetic patients maintain samgue sugar levels. This is very useful for women who have diabetes and have a higher body weight than their standard and thus trying to lose it.

HEALTHY BODY AND LIFESTYLE
Keta lifestyle can be defined as "Healthy". During the basic Keto diet plan, there is an increase in fat intake and reduction in sugar and carbohydrate consumption. Keto diet also helps to reduce the risk of having the so-called "fatty liver disease" and other inflammations, resulting from the consumption of many sweets and otherwise unbalanced and unhealthy diet. Properly following the diet leads your body to be fit and live a healthy lifestyle.

A DEEP SLEEP
Women who follow a keto diet have stated that they feel very satisfied to sleep deeply. Their sleep cycle also improves significantly. After 4 to 5 days of starting the diet, the sleep cycle improves. Feelings of restlessness are reduced and the desire to sleep longer is born. Upon awakening, the body will feel more relaxed and rested.

THE KETO DIET CAN CURE CANCER
The keto diet is also a way to cure very serious diseases among which one of them is cancer. Keto diet helps as stop the growth of tumors. Research has shown that ketone bodies can provide energy to your body without being the food that can feed a cancerous tumor.

REDUCES SUNBURN
The ketogenic diet could become the daily way of life with the benefits it brings. It starts with better control of blood sugar levels which in turn helps reduce "cravings" and the need to eat. So the body can resist longer without the need to eat sugar and sweets. Ketogenic dieting also induces intermittent fasting, which becomes common in women over 50 who follow this type of eating plan.

IMPROVES HEART HEALTH AND SHARPENS THE BRAIN
The ketogenic diet, although high in fat, can also benefit heart function. A year-long study by scientists showed that 22 out of 26 cases of heart disease patients had an improvement in their condition. Finally, particularly for women who experience the keto diet with intermittent fasting, there is evidence of improved brain work. Many trials have shown that this increased efficiency is due to the fact that the brain works better on ketones than on blood sugar.

AIDS DIFFERENT DISEASES
Keto can also help several diseases. It helps to improve your acne, which is normally a big nuisance for women. It is also a cure for polycystic ovary syndrome and nervous system disorders.

IMPROVES NEUROLOGICAL HEALTH
Aging can pose several risks to neurological health, including dementia and Alzheimer's disease. Research shows that this is due to increased blood sugar levels. Keeping this sugar level normal can help your brain work faster and improve your memory. The Keto diet improves your neurological health precisely because of the reduction of sugar in your diet.

As far as weight gain in women aged 50 and older, it must be said that this is common. This can cause some women stress and neurological problems. The keto diet is the behavior way to improve your mental health and live the life you dream of.

FIGHT FATIGUE
Getting older and having a slower metabolism often makes you feel tired. To feel younger and more active at the same time, and fight fatigue, the best way is to exercise, which also helps you lose excess weight. The goal remains first to burn stubborn fats, especially on the belly, abdominal fat leads to visceral fats that compress the internal organs and prevent them from functioning properly.

LOWERS BLOOD PRESSURE

Hypertension is a significant risk factor for many diseases such as kidney failure, stroke and heart disease. The ketogenic diet helps lower blood pressure and prevents the onset of these diseases. The ketogenic diet can help you live longer. With the ketogenic diet, you can lose weight in just a few days by following a proper eating plan. It generally allows the body to work in better condition.

When you reduce carbohydrates, it becomes easier to lose weight in a few days. For women, it is a desire to look nice, beautiful and fit. The keto diet provides a quick and easy to follow program with a low carbohydrate diet that helps you lose weight in a short period, but with long-term benefits.

IMPROVES THE FUNCTIONING OF THE IMMUNE SYSTEM

The keto diet is very also very important for women as it provides them in genele many benefits for their health. Important is the concept of intermittent fasting provided in the ketogenic diet that as far as women are concerned helps them to protect their immune system and to reduce the risk of breast cancer. For women who follow a Keto diet program, the risk of contracting common diseases is also minimized.

HEALS BONE DISEASES

Studies have also shown that women over the age of 50, suffering from arthritis, who follow a specific keto diet with strong reduction in carbohydrates had a strong reduction in pain.

Researchers have shown with several evidences that keto is a very suitable diet for women and especially for women who are over 50 years old. This diet does not create damage to the body and helps to combat the stress of aging, usually present in women facing menopause, making women who practice it feel younger, vital and healthy. It is a complete package that not only protects you from disease, but also gives you the ability to regain energy and maintain your ideal body weight.

SIDE EFFECTS YOU NEED TO KNOW ABOUT KETO DIET

The diet may cause some side effects, including:

INDUCTION INFLUENCE: Symptoms include confusion, clouding of the mind, irritability, lethargy and nausea. These symptoms are common during the first week of the diet.

Treatment: consume salt and water. These symptoms can be cured by introducing enough water and salt into your system. Another even better option, could be drinking broth every day

LEG CRAMPS: Leg cramps are painful.

The cure: take enough salt and drink plenty of fluids. Taking magnesium supplements is also a good idea. Ingesting slow-release magnesium tablets daily during the first three weeks of age is a safe remedy.

CONSTIPATION: Constipation is another side effect of dieting.

The cure: get enough salt and water. Also, include more fiber in your diet, such as fruits and vegetables.

BAD BREATH: Bad breath is another unpleasant problem that can arise.

The cure: eat more carbohydrates. Ingest enough salt and drink enough fluids. Maintain good oral hygiene.

PALPITATIONS

The cure: taking enough fluids is the easiest solution.

In general, you can eliminate all side effects of Keto:

- Drink more water
- Increase your salt intake
- Eat enough fat

BREAKFAST RECIPES

1. *BACON OMELET*

Servings: 3   **Cook Time: 15 Min**   **Prep Time: 10 Min**

INGREDIENTS:

- ✓ 4 large organic eggs
- ✓ 1 tbsp fresh chives, minced
- ✓ Salt and ground black pepper, as required
- ✓ 4 bacon slices
- ✓ 1 tbsp unsalted butter
- ✓ 2 ounces cheddar cheese, shredded

DIRECTIONS:

- ➢ In a bowl, add the eggs, chives, salt and black pepper
- ➢ Beat until well combined.
- ➢ Heat a non-stick frying pan over medium-high heat and cook the bacon slices for about 8–10 minutes.
- ➢ Place the bacon onto a paper towel-lined plate to drain
- ➢ Then chop the bacon slices.
- ➢ With paper towels, wipe out the frying pan.
- ➢ In the same frying pan, melt butter over medium-low heat
- ➢ Cook the egg mixture for about 2 minutes.
- ➢ Carefully flip the omelet and top with chopped bacon
- ➢ Cook for 1–2 minutes or until the desired doneness of eggs.
- ➢ Remove from heat and immediately, place the cheese in the center of the
- ➢ omelet.
- ➢ Fold the edges of the omelet over the cheese and cut it into 2 portions. Serve immediately and enjoy!

NUTRITION INFORMATION: Calories 427 - Carbohydrates 1.2g - Fibers 0g - Fats 1g - Proteins 29.1g

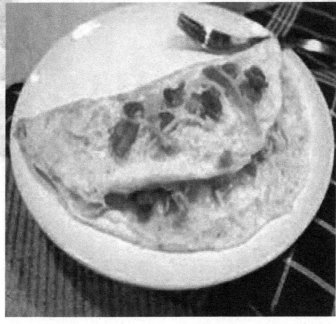

2. *YOGURT WAFFLES*

Servings: 4   **Cook Time: 25 Min**   **Prep Time: 15 Min**

INGREDIENTS:

- ½ cup golden flax seeds meal
- ½ cup plus
- 3 tablespoons almond flour
- 1½ tbsp. granulated erythritol
- 1 tbsp. unsweetened vanilla whey protein powder
- ½ tsp. organic powder
- ¼ tsp. xanthan gum
- Salt, to taste
- 1 large organic egg, white and yolk separated
- 1 organic whole egg
- 2 tbsp. unsweetened almond milk 1½ tbsp. unsalted butter
- 3 oz. plain Greek yogurt
- ¼ tsp. baking soda.

DIRECTIONS:

- Preheat the waffle iron and then grease it.
- In a large bowl, add the flour, erythritol, protein powder, baking soda, baking powder, xanthan gum, salt, and mix until well combined.
- In a second small bowl, add the egg white and beat until stiff peaks form.
- In a third bowl, add 2 egg yolks, whole egg, almond milk, butter, yogurt and beat until well combined.
- Place egg mixture into the bowl of flour mixture and mix until well combined.
- Gently, fold in the beaten egg whites.
- Place ¼ cup of the mixture into preheated waffle iron and cook for about 4–5 minutes or until golden-brown.
- Repeat with the remaining mixture. Serve warm.

NUTRITION INFORMATION: Calories: 250 kcal Carbs: 3.2 g Total Carbs: 8.8 g Fiber: 5.6 g Sugar: 1.3 g Protein 8.4 g.

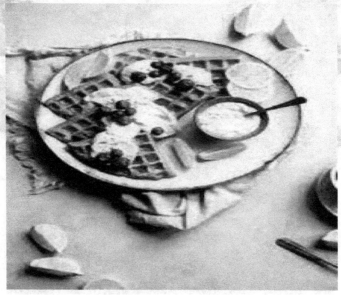

3. *SHEET PAN EGGS WITH VEGGIES AND PARMESAN*

Servings: 4   **Cook Time: 15 Min**   **Prep Time: 5 Min**

INGREDIENTS:

- ✓ 6 large eggs, whisked
- ✓ Salt and pepper
- ✓ 1 small red pepper, diced
- ✓ 1 small yellow onion, chopped
- ✓ 1/2 cup diced mushrooms
- ✓ 1/2 cup diced zucchini
- ✓ 1/3 cup parmesan cheese

DIRECTIONS:

- ➤ Now, preheat the oven to 350°F and grease cooking spray on a rimmed baking sheet.
- ➤ In a cup, whisk the eggs with salt and pepper until sparkling.
- ➤ Remove the peppers, onions, mushrooms, and courgettes until well mixed.
- ➤ Pour the mixture into a baking sheet and scatter over a layer of evenness.
- ➤ Sprinkle with parmesan, and bake until the egg is set for 13 to 16 minutes.
- ➤ Let it cool down slightly, then cut to squares for serving.

NUTRITION INFORMATION: Calories: 180 Fat: 10 g Protein: 14.5 g Carbs: 5 g

4. *ALMOND BUTTER MUFFINS*

Servings: 6   **Cook Time: 25 Min**   **Prep Time: 10 Min**

INGREDIENTS:

- ✓ 1 cups almond flour
- ✓ 1/2 cup powdered erythritol
- ✓ 1 teaspoons baking powder
- ✓ 1/4 tsp. salt
- ✓ 3/4 cup almond butter, warmed
- ✓ 3/4 cup unsweetened oat milk
- ✓ 2 large eggs

DIRECTIONS:

- ➤ Now, preheat the oven to 350°F, and line a paper liner muffin pan.
- ➤ In a mixing bowl, whisk the almond flour and the erythritol, baking powder, and salt.
- ➤ Whisk the oat milk, almond butter, and eggs together in a separate bowl.
- ➤ Drop the wet ingredients into the dry until just mixed together.
- ➤ Spoon the batter into the prepared pan and bake for 22 to 25 minutes until clean comes out the knife inserted in the middle.
- ➤ Cook the muffins in the pan for 5 minutes. Then, switch onto a cooling rack with wire.

NUTRITION INFORMATION: Calories: 135 Fat: 11 g Protein: 6 g Carbs: 4 g

5. SPINACH, MUSHROOM AND GOAT CHEESE FRITTATA

Servings: 5   **Cook Time: 20 Min**   **Prep Time: 15 Min**

INGREDIENTS:

- ✓ 2 tbsp olive oil
- ✓ 1 cup fresh mushrooms, sliced
- ✓ 6 bacon slices, cooked and chopped
- ✓ 1 cup spinach, shredded
- ✓ 10 large eggs, beaten
- ✓ ½ cup goat cheese, crumbled
- ✓ Pepper and salt

DIRECTIONS:

- ➤ Preheat the oven to 350°F.
- ➤ Heat oil and add the mushrooms and fry for 3 minutes until they start to brown, stirring frequently.
- ➤ Fold in the bacon and spinach and cook for about 1 to 2 minutes, or until the spinach is wilted.
- ➤ Slowly pour in the beaten eggs and cook for 3 to 4 minutes
- ➤ Making use of a spatula, lift the edges for allowing uncooked egg to flow underneath.
- ➤ Top with the goat cheese, then sprinkle the salt and pepper to season.
- ➤ Bake in the preheated oven for about 15 minutes until lightly golden brown around the edges.
- ➤ Serve and enjoy!

NUTRITION INFORMATION: Calories 265 Fats 11.6g Fibers 8.6g Carbohydrates 5.1g Proteins 12.9g

6. CLASSIC WESTERN OMELET

Serving: 1   **Cook Time: 10 Min**   **Prep Time: 5 Min**

INGREDIENTS:

- ✓ 2 teaspoons coconut oil
- ✓ 3 large eggs, whisked
- ✓ 1 tbsp. heavy cream
- ✓ Salt and pepper
- ✓ 1/4 cup diced green pepper
- ✓ 1/4 cup diced yellow onion
- ✓ 1/4 cup diced ham

DIRECTIONS:

- ➤ In a small bowl, whisk the eggs, heavy cream, salt, and pepper.
- ➤ Heat up 1 tsp. of coconut oil over medium heat in a small skillet.
- ➤ Add the peppers and onions, then sauté the ham for 3 to 4 minutes.
- ➤ Spoon the mixture in a cup, and heat the skillet with the remaining oil.
- ➤ Pour in the whisked eggs & cook until the egg's bottom begins to set.
- ➤ Tilt the pan and cook until almost set to spread the egg.
- ➤ Spoon the ham and veggie mixture over half of the omelet and turn over.
- ➤ Let cook the omelet until the eggs are set and then serve hot.

NUTRITION INFORMATION: Calories: 415 Fat: 32,5 g Protein: 5 g Carbs: 6,5 g

7. BROCCOLI MUFFINS

Servings: 5   **Cook Time: 20 Min**   **Prep Time: 15 Min**

INGREDIENTS:

- ✓ 2 tbsp. unsalted butter
- ✓ 6 large organic eggs
- ✓ ½ cup heavy whipping cream
- ✓ ½ cup Parmesan cheese, grated
- ✓ Salt and ground black pepper, to taste
- ✓ 1¼ cup broccoli, chopped
- ✓ 2 tbsp. fresh parsley, chopped
- ✓ ½ cup Swiss cheese, grated.

DIRECTIONS:

- ➢ Preheat your oven to 350°F. Grease a 12-cup muffin tin.
- ➢ In a bowl, add the eggs, cream, Parmesan cheese, salt, black pepper and beat until well combined.
- ➢ Divide the broccoli and parsley in the bottom of each prepared muffin cup evenly.
- ➢ Top with the egg mixture, followed by the Swiss cheese.
- ➢ Bake for about 20 minutes, rotating the pan once halfway through.
- ➢ Remove from the oven and place onto a wire rack for about 5 minutes before serving.
- ➢ Carefully, invert the muffins onto a serving platter and serve warm.

NUTRITION INFORMATION: Calories: 231 kcal Total Carbs: 2.5 g Fiber: 0.5 g Sugar: 0.9 g Protein: 13.5 g.

8. GREEN VEGETABLES QUICHE

Servings: 4   **Cook Time: 20 Min**   **Prep Time: 20 Min**

INGREDIENTS:

- ✓ 6 organic eggs
- ✓ ½ cup unsweetened almond milk
- ✓ Salt and ground black pepper, as required
- ✓ 2 cups fresh baby spinach, chopped
- ✓ ½ cup green bell pepper, seeded and chopped
- ✓ 1 scallion, chopped
- ✓ ¼ cup fresh cilantro, chopped
- ✓ 1 tbsp fresh chives, minced
- ✓ 3 tbsp mozzarella cheese, grated

DIRECTIONS:

- ➢ Preheat your oven to 400°F. Lightly grease a pie dish.
- ➢ In a bowl, add eggs, almond milk, salt and black pepper. Beat until well combined. Set aside.
- ➢ In another bowl, add the vegetables and herbs and mix well.
- ➢ At the bottom of the prepared pie dish, place the veggie mixture evenly and top with the egg mixture.
- ➢ Let the quiche bake for about 20 minutes.
- ➢ Remove the pie dish from the oven and immediately sprinkle with the Parmesan cheese.
- ➢ Set aside for about 5 minutes before slicing. Cut into desired sized wedges.
- ➢ Serve warm and enjoy!

NUTRITION INFORMATION: Calories 298 Fats 10.4g Fibers 5.9g Carbohydrates 4.1g Proteins 7.9g

9. SHEET PAN EGGS WITH HAM AND PEPPER JACK

Servings: 6   **Cook Time: 15 Min**   **Prep Time: 5 Min**

INGREDIENTS:
- ✓ 12 large eggs, whisked
- ✓ Salt and pepper
- ✓ 2 cups diced ham
- ✓ Oat milk

DIRECTIONS:
- ➤ Now, preheat the oven to 350°F and grease a rimmed baking sheet with cooking spray.
- ➤ Whisk the eggs in a mixing bowl then add salt and pepper until frothy.
- ➤ Stir in the ham and oat milk and mix until well combined.
- ➤ Pour the mixture into baking sheets and spread it into an even layer.
- ➤ Bake for 12 to 15 mins until the egg is set.
- ➤ Let cool slightly then cut it into squares to serve.

NUTRITION INFORMATION: Calories: 235 Fat: 15g Protein: 21g Carbs: 2.5g

10. BACON & AVOCADO OMELET

Servings: 1   **Cook Time: 5 Min**   **Prep Time: 5 Min**

INGREDIENTS:
- ✓ 1 slice crispy bacon
- ✓ 2 large organic eggs
- ✓ 5 cup freshly grated Parmesan cheese
- ✓ 2 tbsp Ghee or coconut oil or butter
- ✓ Half small avocado

DIRECTIONS:
- ➤ Prepare the bacon to your liking and set aside.
- ➤ Combine the eggs, Parmesan cheese and your choice of finely chopped herbs.
- ➤ Warm a skillet and add the butter/ghee to melt using the medium-high heat setting. When the pan is hot, whisk and add the eggs.
- ➤ Prepare the omelet working it towards the middle of the pan for about 30 seconds. When firm, flip, and cook it for another 30 seconds.
- ➤ Arrange the omelet on a plate and garnish with the crunched bacon bits. Serve with sliced avocado.
- ➤ Enjoy!

NUTRITION INFORMATION: Calories 719 - Carbohydrates 3.3g - Proteins 30g - Fats 63g

11. PUMPKIN BREAD

Servings: 5   **Cook Time: 1 H**   **Prep Time: 15 Min**

INGREDIENTS:
- ✓ 1 ⅔ cup almond flour
- ✓ 1½ tsp. organic baking powder
- ✓ ½ tsp. pumpkin pie spice
- ✓ ½ tsp. ground cinnamon
- ✓ ½ tsp. ground cloves
- ✓ ½ tsp. salt
- ✓ 8 oz. cream cheese, softened
- ✓ 6 organic eggs, divided
- ✓ 1 tbsp. coconut flour
- ✓ 1 cup powdered erythritol, divided
- ✓ 1 tsp. stevia powder, divided
- ✓ 1 tsp. organic lemon extract
- ✓ 1 cup homemade pumpkin puree
- ✓ ½ cup coconut oil, melted

DIRECTIONS:
- ➤ Preheat your oven to 325°F. Lightly, grease 2 bread loaf pans.
- ➤ In a bowl, place almond flour, baking powder, spices, salt and mix until well combined.
- ➤ In a second bowl, add the cream cheese, 1 egg, coconut flour
- ➤ Then ¼ cup of erythritol, ¼ teaspoon of the stevia and with a wire whisk, beat until smooth.
- ➤ In a third bowl, add the pumpkin puree, oil, 5 eggs, ¾ cup of the erythritol, ¾ teaspoon of the stevia, and with a wire whisk, beat until well combined.
- ➤ Add the pumpkin mixture into the bowl of the flour mixture and mix until just combined.
- ➤ Place about ¼ of the pumpkin mixture into each loaf pan evenly.
- ➤ Top each pan with the cream cheese mixture evenly, followed by the remaining pumpkin mixture.
- ➤ Bake for about 50–60 minutes or until a toothpick inserted in the center comes out clean.
- ➤ Remove the bread pans from oven and place onto a wire rack and let it be for 10 minutes.
- ➤ With a sharp knife, cut each bread loaf in the desired-sized slices and serve.

NUTRITION INFORMATION: Calories: 216 kcal | Total Carbs: 4.5 g | Fiber: 2 g | Sugar: 1.1 g | Protein: 3.4 g.

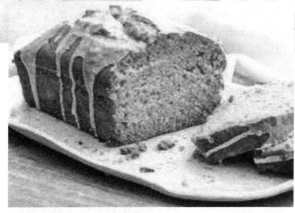

12. *CHEDDAR SCRAMBLE*

Servings: 2 **Cook Time: 8 Min** **Prep Time: 10 Min**

INGREDIENTS:

- ✓ 2 tbsp olive oil
- ✓ 1 small yellow onion, chopped finely
- ✓ 12 large organic eggs, beaten lightly
- ✓ Salt and ground black pepper, as required
- ✓ 4 ounces cheddar cheese, shredded

DIRECTIONS:

- ➤ In a large wok, heat oil over medium heat and sauté the onion for about 4–5 minutes.
- ➤ Add the eggs, salt and black pepper and cook for about 3 minutes, stirring continuously.
- ➤ Remove from the heat and immediately, stir in the cheese. Serve immediately and enjoy!

NUTRITION INFORMATION: Calories 264 Carbohydrates 2.1g Fibers 0.3g Fats 1.4g Proteins 17.4g

13. *CHICKEN & ASPARAGUS FRITTATA*

Servings: 4 **Cook Time: 12 Min** **Prep Time: 15 Min**

INGREDIENTS:

- ✓ ½ cup grass-fed cooked chicken breast, chopped
- ✓ ⅓ cup Parmesan cheese, grated
- ✓ 6 organic eggs, beaten lightly
- ✓ Salt and ground black pepper, as required
- ✓ ⅓ cup boiled asparagus, chopped
- ✓ ¼ cup cherry tomatoes, halved
- ✓ ¼ cup mozzarella cheese, shredded

DIRECTIONS:

Preheat the broiler of the oven.

- ➤ In a bowl, add the Parmesan cheese, eggs, salt and black pepper. Beat until
- ➤ well combined.
- ➤ In a large ovenproof wok, melt butter over medium-high heat and cook the chicken and asparagus for about 2–3 minutes.
- ➤ Add the egg mixture and tomatoes and stir to combine. Cook for about 4–5 minutes.
- ➤ Remove from the heat and sprinkle with the Parmesan cheese.
- ➤ Now, transfer the wok under the broiler and broil for about 3–4 minutes or until slightly puffed.
- ➤ Cut into desired sized wedges and serve immediately. Enjoy!

NUTRITION INFORMATION: Calories 158 - Carbohydrates 1.7g - Fibers 0.4g - Fats 1g - Proteins 20g

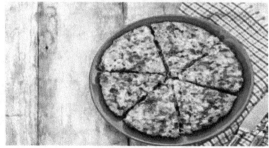

14. SPINACH ARTICHOKE BREAKFAST BAKE

Servings: 7   **Cook Time: 20 Min**   **Prep Time: 15 Min**

INGREDIENTS:

- ✓ ¼ cup milk, fat-free
- ✓ ¼ tsp. ground pepper
- ✓ ⅓ cup red pepper, diced
- ✓ ½ cup feta cheese crumbles
- ✓ ½ cup scallions, finely sliced
- ✓ ¾ cup canned artichokes, chopped, drained, & patted dry
- ✓ 1¼ tsp. kosher salt
- ✓ 1 clove garlic, minced
- ✓ 1 tbsp. dill, chopped
- ✓ 10 oz. spinach, frozen, chopped & drained
- ✓ 2 tbsp. parmesan cheese, grated
- ✓ 4 large egg whites
- ✓ 8 large eggs.

DIRECTIONS:

- ➢ Preheat the oven to 375°F and grease a large baking dish with nonstick spray or preferred fat source.
- ➢ In a small bowl, combine the spinach, artichoke, scallions, garlic, red pepper, and fill.
- ➢ Combine completely and then pour into the baking dish, spreading into an even layer.
- ➢ In a mixing bowl, combine eggs, egg whites, salt, pepper, parmesan, and milk.
- ➢ Whisk until completely combined, then add feta and mix once more. Pour the egg mixture evenly over the vegetables in the baking dish.
- ➢ Bake for about 35 minutes, until a butter knife inserted in the center comes out clean.
- ➢ Allow to cool for about 10 minutes before cutting into eight equal pieces. Serve warm!

NUTRITION INFORMATION: Calories: 574 kcal Carbs: 2 g Fiber: 0.7 g Sugar: 0.1 g Protein: 47 g Fat: 54 g Sodium: 254 mg.

15. BERRY CHOCOLATE BREAKFAST BOWL

Servings: 2   **Cook Time: 0 Min**   **Prep Time: 10 Min**

INGREDIENTS:

- ✓ ½ cup strawberries, fresh or frozen
- ✓ ½ cup blueberries, fresh or frozen
- ✓ 1 cup unsweetened almond milk
- ✓ Sugar-free maple syrup to taste
- ✓ 2 tbsp unsweetened cocoa powder
- ✓ 1 tbsp cashew nuts for topping

DIRECTIONS:

- ➢ The berries must be divided into four bowls, pour on the almond milk.
- ➢ Drizzle with the maple syrup and sprinkle the cocoa powder on top, a tbsp per bowl.
- ➢ Top with the cashew nuts and enjoy immediately.

NUTRITION INFORMATION: Calories 287 Fats 5.9g Fibers 11.4g Carbohydrates 3.1g Proteins 4.2g

16. SALMON WITH CHILI-GARLIC

Servings: 4   Cook Time: 15 Min   Prep Time: 10 Min

INGREDIENTS:

- ✓ 5 tbsp sweet chili sauce
- ✓ ¼ cup coconut aminos
- ✓ 4 salmon fillets
- ✓ 3 tbsp green onions, chopped
- ✓ 3 cloves garlic, peeled and minced

DIRECTIONS:

- ➤ In a large saucepan, place a trivet and pour a cup or two of water into the pan. Bring to a boil.
- ➤ In a small bowl, whisk well sweet chili sauce, garlic, and coconut aminos.
- ➤ Place salmon in a heatproof dish that fits inside a saucepan. Season salmon with pepper. Drizzle with sweet chili sauce mixture. Sprinkle green onions on top of the filet.
- ➤ Seal dish with foil. Place the dish on the trivet inside the saucepan. Cover and steam for 15 minutes.
- ➤ Serve and enjoy!

NUTRITION INFORMATION: Calories 409 Fats 14.4g Carbohydrates 0.9g- Proteins 65.4g

17. CAULIFLOWER & MUSHROOM RISOTTO

Servings: 4   Cook Time: 10 Min   Prep Time: 5 Min

INGREDIENTS:

- ✓ 1 grated head of cauliflower
- ✓ 1 cup vegetable stock
- ✓ 9 oz. chopped mushrooms
- ✓ 2 tbsp. butter
- ✓ 1 cup coconut cream

DIRECTIONS:

- ➤ Pour the stock in a saucepan. Boil and set aside.
- ➤ Prepare a skillet with butter and sauté the mushrooms until golden. Grate and stir in the cauliflower and stock.
- ➤ Simmer and add the cream, cooking until the cauliflower is al dente.
- ➤ Serve.

NUTRITION INFORMATION: Calories: 186 kcal Carbs: 4 g Protein: 1 g Fats: 17 g.

18. PITA PIZZA

Servings: 2   Cook Time: 10 Min   Prep Time: 15 Min

INGREDIENTS:

- ✓ ½ cup marinara sauce
- ✓ 1 low-carb pita
- ✓ 1 oz. cheddar cheese
- ✓ 14 slices pepperoni
- ✓ 1 oz. roasted red peppers.

DIRECTIONS:

- ➤ Program the oven temperature setting to 450°F.
- ➤ Slice the pita in half and place onto a foil-lined baking tray. Rub with a bit of oil and toast for one to two minutes.
- ➤ Pour the sauce over the bread.
- ➤ Sprinkle using the cheese and other toppings. Bake until the cheese melts (5 minutes).
- ➤ Cool thoroughly.

NUTRITION INFORMATION: Calories: 250 kcal Carbs: 4 g Protein: 13 g Fats: 19 g.

19. BRAISED CHICKEN IN ITALIAN TOMATO SAUCE

Servings: 4   **Cook Time: 4 H**   **Prep Time: 15 Min**

INGREDIENTS:

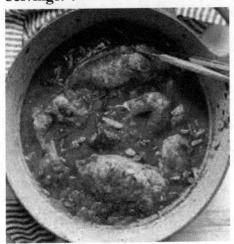

- ✓ 1/4 cup olive oil, divided
- ✓ 4 (4-ounce/113-g) boneless chicken thighs
- ✓ Pepper and salt
- ✓ 1/2 cup chicken stock
- ✓ 4 ounces (113 g) julienned oil-packed sun-dried tomatoes
- ✓ 1 (28-ounce/794-g) can sodium-free diced tomatoes
- ✓ 2 tbsps. dried oregano
- ✓ 2 tbsps. minced garlic
- ✓ Red pepper flakes, to taste
- ✓ 2 tbsps. chopped fresh parsley

DIRECTIONS:

- ➤ Heat oil then put the chicken thighs in the skillet and sprinkle salt and black pepper to season.
- ➤ Sear the chicken thighs for 10 minutes or until well browned.
- ➤ Flip them halfway through the cooking time.
- ➤ Put the chicken thighs, stock, tomatoes, oregano, garlic, and red pepper flakes into the slow cooker. Stir to coat the chicken thighs well.
- ➤ High cook for 4 hrs.
- ➤ Transfer the chicken thighs to four plates.
- ➤ Pour the sauce which remains in the slow cooker over the chicken thighs and top with fresh parsley before serving warm.

NUTRITION INFORMATION: Calories: 464 Fat: 12.1g Carbs: 6.4 g Protein: 13.1g

20. STEAMED COD WITH GINGER

Servings: 4   **Cook Time: 15 Min**   **Prep Time: 15 Min**

INGREDIENTS:

- ✓ 4 cod fillets, skin removed
- ✓ 3 tbsp lemon juice, freshly squeezed
- ✓ 2 tbsp coconut aminos
- ✓ 2 tbsp grated ginger 6 scallions, chopped

DIRECTIONS:

- ➤ In a large saucepan, place a trivet and pour a cup or two of water into the pan
- ➤ Bring to a boil.
- ➤ In a small bowl, whisk well lemon juice, coconut aminos, coconut oil and grated ginger.
- ➤ Place scallions in a heatproof dish that fits inside a saucepan.
- ➤ Season scallion's mon with pepper and salt
- ➤ rizzle with ginger mixture. Sprinkle scallions on top.
- ➤ Seal dish with foil. Place the dish on the trivet inside the saucepan
- ➤ Cover and steam for 15 minutes.
- ➤ Serve and enjoy!

NUTRITION INFORMATION: Calories 514 - Fats 40g - Carbohydrates 10g - Proteins 28.3g

21. ITALIAN STYLE HALIBUT PACKETS

Servings: 4   **Cook Time: 20 Min**   **Prep Time: 10 Min**

INGREDIENTS:

- ✓ 1 cups cauliflower florets
- ✓ 1 cup roasted red pepper strips
- ✓ ½ cup sliced sun-dried tomatoes
- ✓ 4 (4-ounce) halibut fillets
- ✓ ¼ cup chopped fresh basil
- ✓ 1 lemon juice
- ✓ ¼ cup good-quality olive oil
- ✓ Sea salt, for seasoning
- ✓ Freshly ground black pepper, for seasoning.

DIRECTIONS:

➤ Preheat the oven. Set the oven temperature to 400°F. Make the packets.

➤ Divide the cauliflower, red pepper strips, and sun-dried tomato between the four pieces of foil, placing the vegetables in the middle of each piece.

➤ Top each pile with one halibut fillet and top each fillet with equal amounts of the basil, lemon juice, and olive oil.

➤ Fold and crimp the foil to form sealed packets of fish and vegetables and place them on the baking sheet.

➤ Bake the packets for about 20 minutes, until the fish flakes with a fork. Be careful of the steam when you open the packet!

➤ Transfer the vegetables and halibut to four plates, season with salt and pepper, and serve immediately.

NUTRITION INFORMATION: Calories: 313 kcal Fat: 14.1 g Carbs: 3.2 g Fiber: 10.4 g Protein: 15.4 g.

22. STEAMED COD WITH GINGER

Servings: 4   **Cook Time: 15 Min**   **Prep Time: 10 Min**

INGREDIENTS:

- ✓ 4 flounder fillets
- ✓ 1 tbsp chopped fresh dill
- ✓ 2 tbsp capers, chopped
- ✓ 4 lemon wedges

DIRECTIONS:

➤ In a large saucepan, place a trivet and pour a cup or two of water into the pan. Bring to a boil.

➤ Place flounder in a heatproof dish that fits inside a saucepan. Season flounder with pepper and salt. Drizzle with olive oil on all sides. Sprinkle dill and capers on top of the filet.

➤ Seal dish with foil. Place the dish on the trivet inside the saucepan

➤ Cover and steam for 15 minutes.

➤ Serve and enjoy with lemon wedges.

NUTRITION INFORMATION: Calories 447 Fats 35.9g Carbohydrates 8.6g Proteins 20.3g

23. *CHEESY ROASTED CHICKEN*

Servings: 6 **Cook Time: 10 Min** **Prep Time: 15 Min**

INGREDIENTS:

✓ 3 cups of chopped roasted chicken

DIRECTIONS:

➢ Oven: 350F
➢ Be sure to rub butter or spray with non-stick cooking spray. Put in the chicken and toss thoroughly.
➢ Be sure to leave space between piles.
➢ Bake for 4-6 minutes. The moment they turn golden brown at the edges, take them off.
➢ Serve hot.

NUTRITION INFORMATION: Calories: 387 Fat: 19.5g Carbs: 3.9 g Protein: 14.5g

24. *MEATBALLS SALAD*

Servings: 4 **Cook Time: 10 Min** **Prep Time: 10 Min**

INGREDIENTS:

✓ 1-pound (454 g) ground beef
✓ ¼ cup pork rinds, crushed
✓ 1 egg, whisked
✓ 1 onion, grated
✓ 1 tbsp fresh parsley, chopped

SALAD:

✓ 1 cup chopped arugula
✓ 1 cucumber, sliced
✓ 1 cup cherry tomatoes, halved

✓ ½ tsp dried oregano
✓ 1 garlic clove, minced
✓ Salt and black pepper to taste
✓ 2 tbsp olive oil, divided

✓ 1½ tbsp lemon juice
✓ Salt and pepper to taste

DIRECTIONS:

➢ Stir together the beef, pork rinds, whisked egg, onion, parsley, oregano
➢ Add garlic, salt and pepper in a large bowl until completely mixed.
➢ On a lightly floured surface, using a cookie scoop to scoop out equal-sized amounts of the beef mixture and form into meatballs with your palm.
➢ Heat 1 tbsp olive oil in a large skillet over medium heat, fry the meatballs for about 4 minutes on each side until cooked through.
➢ Remove from the heat and set aside on a plate to cool.
➢ In a salad bowl, mix the arugula, cucumber, cherry tomatoes, 1 tbsp olive oil, and lemon juice. Season with salt and pepper.
➢ In a third bowl, whisk the almond milk, yogurt, and mint until well blended. Pour the mixture over the salad. Serve topped with the meatballs. Enjoy!

NUTRITION INFORMATION: Calories 302 Fats 13g Carbohydrates 6g Proteins 7g Fibers 4g

25. TURKEY BREAST WITH TOMATO-OLIVE SALSA

Servings: 4 **Cook Time: 10 Min** **Prep Time: 20 Min**

INGREDIENTS:
FOR TURKEY:
- ✓ 4 boneless turkey, skinned.
- ✓ 3 tbsps. olive oil
- ✓ Salt
- ✓ Pepper

FOR SALSA:
- ➤ 6 chopped tomatoes
- ➤ 5 ounces of pitted and chopped olives
- ➤ 2 crushed garlic cloves
- ➤ Pepper
- ➤ Salt

DIRECTIONS:
- ➤ In a bowl, put salt, pepper, and three spoons of oil, mix and coat the turkey with this mixture.
- ➤ Place it on a preheated grill and grill for ten minutes.
- ➤ In another bowl, mix garlic, olives, tomatoes, pepper, and drop the rest of the oil
- ➤ Sprinkle salt and toss. Serve this salsa with turkey is warm.

NUTRITION INFORMATION: Calories: 387 Fat: 12.5g Carbs: 3.1 g Protein: 18.6g

26. TACO CASSEROLE

Servings: 8 **Cook Time: 20 Min** **Prep Time: 10 Min**

INGREDIENTS:
- ✓ 1½ to 2 lb. ground turkey or beef
- ✓ 2 tbsp. taco seasoning
- ✓ 8 oz. shredded cheddar cheese
- ✓ 1 cup salsa
- ✓ 16 oz. cottage cheese.

DIRECTIONS:
- ➤ Heat the oven to reach 400 °F.
- ➤ Combine the taco seasoning and ground meat in a casserole dish.
- ➤ Bake it for 20 minutes.
- ➤ Combine the salsa and both kinds of cheese. Set aside for now.
- ➤ Carefully transfer the casserole dish from the oven.
- ➤ Drain away the cooking juices from the meat.
- ➤ Break the meat into small pieces and mash with a masher or fork.
- ➤ Sprinkle with cheese.
- ➤ Bake in the oven for 15 to 20 more minutes until the top is browned.

NUTRITION INFORMATION: Calories: 367 kcal Carbs: 6 g Protein: 45 g Fats: 18 g.

27. CHICKEN, BACON AND AVOCADO CLOUD SANDWICHES

Servings: 6   **Cook Time: 25 Min**   **Prep Time: 10 Min**

INGREDIENTS:

FOR CLOUD BREAD:
- ✓ 3 large eggs
- ✓ 4 oz cream cheese
- ✓ ½ tbsp ground psyllium husk powder

FOR THE SANDWICH:
- ✓ 6 slices of bacon, cooked and chopped
- ✓ 6 slices Pepper Jack cheese
- ✓ ½ avocado, sliced

- ✓ ½ tsp baking powder
- ✓ A pinch of salt

- ✓ 1 cup cooked chicken breasts, shredded
- ✓ 3 tbsp mayo

DIRECTIONS:

- ➢ Preheat oven to 300°F.
- ➢ Prepare a baking sheet by lining it with parchment paper.
- ➢ Separate the egg whites and egg yolks and place into separate bowls
- ➢ Whisk the egg whites until very stiff and set aside.
- ➢ Combine the egg yolks and the cream cheese.
- ➢ Add the psyllium husk powder and baking powder to the egg yolk mixture
- ➢ Then the egg whites into the egg mixture and gently fold in.
- ➢ Dollop the mixture onto the prepared baking sheet to create 12 cloud bread. Use a spatula to gently spread the circles around to form ½-inch thick pieces.
- ➢ Bake for 25 minutes or until the tops are golden brown.
- ➢ Allow the cloud bread to cool completely before serving.
- ➢ an be refrigerated for up to 3 days or frozen for up to 3 months
- ➢ If food prepping, place a layer of parchment paper between each bread slice to avoid having them getting stuck together
- ➢ Simply toast in the oven for 5 minutes when it is time to servings.
- ➢ To assemble sandwiches, place mayonnaise on one side of one cloud bread
- ➢ Layer with the remaining sandwich ingredients and top with another slice of cloud bread
- ➢ Serve and enjoy!

NUTRITION INFORMATION: Calories 333 - Carbohydrates 5g - Fats 26g - Proteins 19.9g

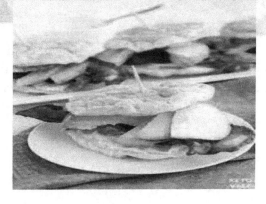

28. CHEESY BACON RANCH CHICKEN

Servings: 8   **Cook Time: 35 Min**   **Prep Time: 40 Min**

INGREDIENTS:

- ✓ 8 boneless and skinned chicken breasts
- ✓ 1 cup of olive oil
- ✓ 8 thick slices of bacon
- ✓ 3 cups of shredded mozzarella
- ✓ 1 1/4 tbsp. of ranch seasoning
- ✓ Chopped chives
- ✓ Kosher salt or pink salt
- ✓ Black pepper

DIRECTIONS:

- ➤ Preheat skillet and heat little oil, and cook bacon evenly on both sides.
- ➤ Save four tbsps. Of drippings and put the others away.
- ➤ Add in salt and pepper in a bowl and rub it over chicken to season.
- ➤ Put 1/2 oil on the flame to cook the chicken from each side for 5 to 7 minutes.
- ➤ When ready, reduce the heat and put in the ranch seasoning, then add mozzarella.
- ➤ Cover and cook on a low flame for 3-5 minutes.
- ➤ Put in bacon fat and chopped chives, then bacon and cover it.
- ➤ Take off and serve warm.

NUTRITION INFORMATION: Calories: 387 Fat: 15.1g Carbs: 5.9 g Protein: 12.9g

29. ROASTED LEMON CHICKEN SANDWICH

Servings: 12   **Cook Time: 1 H 30 Min**   **Prep Time: 15 Min**

INGREDIENTS:

- ✓ 1 kg whole chicken
- ✓ 5 tbsp butter
- ✓ 1 lemon cut into wedges
- ✓ 1 tbsp garlic powder
- ✓ Salt and pepper to taste
- ✓ 2 tbsp mayo
- ✓ Keto-friendly bread

DIRECTIONS:

- ➤ Preheat the oven to 350°F.
- ➤ Grease a deep baking dish with butter.
- ➤ Ensure that the chicken is patted dry and that the gizzards have been removed.
- ➤ Combine the butter, garlic powder, salt and pepper.
- ➤ Rub the entire chicken with it, including in the cavity.
- ➤ Place the lemon and onion inside the chicken and place the chicken in the prepared baking dish.
- ➤ Bake for about 1½ hours, depending on the size of the chicken.
- ➤ Baste the chicken often with the drippings. If the drippings begin to dry, add water.
- ➤ The chicken is done when a thermometer, insert it into the thickest part of the thigh reads 165 degrees F or when the clear juices run when the thickest part of the thigh is pierced.
- ➤ Allow the chicken to cool before slicing.
- ➤ To assemble the sandwich, shred some of the breast meat and mix with the mayonnaise. Place the mixture between the two bread slices. Serve and enjoy!
- ➤ To save the chicken, refrigerated for up to 5 days or freeze for up to 1 month.

NUTRITION INFORMATION: Calories 214 Carbohydrates 1.6g Fats 11.8g Proteins 24.4g

30. BEEF WELLINGTON

Servings: 4   **Cook Time: 40 Min**   **Prep Time: 20 Min**

INGREDIENTS:

- ✓ 2 (4-ounce) grass-fed beef tenderloin steaks, halved
- ✓ Salt and ground black pepper, as required
- ✓ 1 tbsp. butter
- ✓ 1 cup mozzarella cheese, shredded
- ✓ ½ cup almond flour
- ✓ 4 tbsp. liver pate.

DIRECTIONS:

- ➢ Preheat your oven to 400°F. Grease a baking sheet.
- ➢ Season the steaks with pepper and salt.
- ➢ Sear the beef steaks for about 2–3 minutes per side.
- ➢ In a microwave-safe bowl, add the mozzarella cheese and microwave for about 1 minute.
- ➢ Remove from the microwave and stir in the almond flour until a dough forms.
- ➢ Place the dough between 2 parchment paper pieces and, with a rolling pin, roll to flatten it.
- ➢ Remove the upper parchment paper piece. Divide the rolled dough into four pieces.
- ➢ Place one tablespoon of pate onto each dough piece and top with one steak piece.
- ➢ Cover each steak piece with dough completely.
- ➢ Arrange the covered steak pieces onto the prepared baking sheet in a single layer.
- ➢ Baking time: 20-30 minutes. Serve warm.

NUTRITION INFORMATION: Calories: 412 kcal Fat: 15.6g Carbs: 4.9 g Fiber: 9.1g Protein: 18.5g.

31. GARLIC & THYME LAMB CHOPS

Servings: 6   **Cook Time: 10 Min**   **Prep Time: 15 Min**

INGREDIENTS:

- ✓ 6 - 4 oz. lamb chops
- ✓ 4 cloves whole garlic
- ✓ 2 sprigs thyme
- ✓ 1 tsp ground thyme
- ✓ 3 tbsp olive oil

DIRECTIONS:

- ➢ Warm-up a skillet. Put the olive oil. Rub the chops with the spices
- ➢ Put the chops in the skillet with the garlic and sprigs of thyme.
- ➢ Sauté within 3 to 4 minutes. Serve and enjoy!

NUTRITION INFORMATION: Calories 252 Carbohydrates 1g Proteins 14g Fats 21g

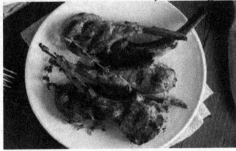

32. INDIAN BUTTERED CHICKEN

Servings: 4   **Cook Time: 30 Min**   **Prep Time: 15 Min**

INGREDIENTS:

- ✓ 3 tbsps. unsalted butter
- ✓ 1 medium yellow onion, chopped
- ✓ 2 garlic cloves, minced
- ✓ 1 tsp. fresh ginger, minced
- ✓ 1 1/2 pounds grass-fed chicken breasts, cut into 3/4-inch chunks
- ✓ 2 tomatoes, chopped finely
- ✓ 1 tbsp. garam masala
- ✓ 1 tsp. red chili powder
- ✓ 1 tsp. ground cumin
- ✓ Salt and ground black pepper, as required
- ✓ 1 cup heavy cream
- ✓ 2 tbsps. fresh cilantro, chopped

DIRECTIONS:

- ➤ In a wok, melt butter and sauté the onions for about 5–6 minutes.
- ➤ Now, add in ginger and garlic and sauté for about 1 minute.
- ➤ Add the tomatoes and cook for about 2–3 minutes, crushing with the back of the spoon.
- ➤ Stir in the chicken, spices, salt, and black pepper, and cook for about 6– 8 minutes or until the desired doneness of the chicken.
- ➤ Put in the cream and cook for about 8–10 more minutes, stirring occasionally.
- ➤ Garnish with fresh cilantro and serve hot.

NUTRITION INFORMATION: Calories: 456 Fat: 14.1g Carbs: 6.8 g Protein: 12.8 g

33. JAMAICAN JERK PORK ROAST

Servings: 12   **Cook Time: 4 H Min**   **Prep Time: 15 Min**

INGREDIENTS:

- ✓ 1 tbsp olive oil
- ✓ 4 lb. pork shoulder
- ✓ ½ cup beef broth
- ✓ 0.25 cup Jamaican Jerk spice blend

DIRECTIONS:

- ➤ Rub the roast well the oil and the jerk spice blend
- ➤ Sear the roast on all sides. Put the beef broth.
- ➤ Simmer within four hours on low. Shred and serve. Enjoy!

NUTRITION INFORMATION: Calories 282 Carbohydrates 0g Proteins 23g Fats 20g

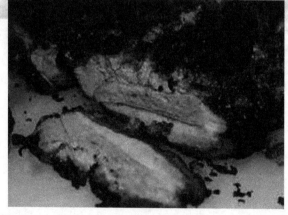

34. BEANS AND SAUSAGE

Servings: 2 **Cook Time: 6Min** **Prep Time: 5 Min**

INGREDIENTS:
- ✓ 4 oz. green beans
- ✓ 4 oz. chicken sausage, sliced
- ✓ 1/2 tsp. dried basil

SEASONING:
- ✓ 1 tbsp. avocado oil
- ✓ 1/4 tsp. salt

- ✓ 1/2 tsp. dried oregano
- ✓ 1/3 cup chicken broth, from chicken sausage

- ✓ 1/8 tsp. ground black pepper

DIRECTIONS:
- ➢ Turn on the instant pot, place all the ingredients in its inner pot and shut with lid, in the sealed position.

- ➢ Press the "manual" button, cook for 6 minutes at high-pressure settings and, when done, do a quick pressure release.
- ➢ Serve immediately.

NUTRITION INFORMATION: Calories: 151 Fats 9.4 g Protein: 11.7 g Carbs: 3.4 g

35. KETO MEATBALLS

Servings: 10 **Cook Time: 20 Min** **Prep Time: 15 Min**

INGREDIENTS:
- ✓ 1 egg
- ✓ 0.5 cup grated Parmesan
- ✓ 0.5 cup shredded mozzarella

- ✓ 1 lb. ground beef
- ✓ 1 tbsp garlic

DIRECTIONS:
- ➢ Warm-up the oven to reach 400°F.
- ➢ Combine all the fixings in a large mixing bowl.

- ➢ Shape into meatballs.
- ➢ Bake within 18-20 minutes. Cool and serve. Enjoy!

NUTRITION INFORMATION: Calories 153 - Carbohydrates 0.7g - Proteins 12.2g - Fats 10.9g

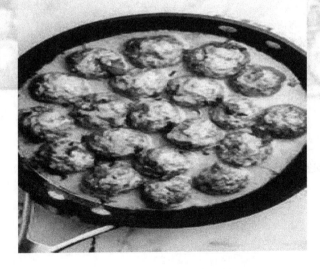

36. KETO CROQUE MONSIEUR

Servings: 2   **Cook Time: 7 Min**   **Prep Time: 5 Min**

INGREDIENTS:

- ✓ 1 eggs
- ✓ ¾ oz. of grated cheese
- ✓ ¾ oz. of ham
- ✓ 1 large slice
- ✓ 3 tbsp. of cream
- ✓ 2 tbsp. of mascarpone 1 oz. of butter
- ✓ Pepper and salt
- ✓ Basil leaves, optional, to garnish.

DIRECTIONS:

- ➤ Carefully crack eggs in a neat bowl, add some salt and pepper. Add the cream, mascarpone, grated cheese, and stir together.
- ➤ Melt the butter over medium heat. The butter must not turn brown. Once the butter has melted, set the heat to low.
- ➤ Add half of the omelette mixture to the frying pan and then immediately place the slice of ham on it.
- ➤ Now pour the rest of the omelette mixture over the ham and then immediately put a lid on it.
- ➤ Allow it to fry for 2-3 minutes over low heat until the top is slightly firmer
- ➤ Slide the omelette onto the lid to turn the omelette.
- ➤ Then put the omelette back in the frying pan to fry for another 1-2 minutes on the other side (still on low heat), then put the lid back on the pan
- ➤ Don't let the omelette cook for too long!
- ➤ It does not matter if it is still liquid.
- ➤ Garnish with a few basil leaves if necessary.

NUTRITION INFORMATION: Calories: 479 kcal Protein: 16 g Fats: 45 g Carbs: 4 g.

37. LOW CARB BROCCOLI LEEK SOUP

Servings: 2   **Cook Time: 15 Min**   **Prep Time: 15 Min**

INGREDIENTS:

- ✓ ½ leek
- ✓ 100 g cream cheese
- ✓ 150 g broccoli
- ✓ ½ cup heavy cream
- ✓ 1 cup of water
- ✓ ¼ tbsp black pepper
- ✓ ½ vegetable bouillon cube
- ✓ ¼ cup basil
- ✓ 1 tsp garlic
- ✓ Salt

DIRECTIONS:

- ➤ Put water into a pan and put broccoli chopped, leek chopped and salt
- ➤ Bring to a boil.
- ➤ Put the remaining ingredients, simmer on low for 1 minute. Remove from heat.
- ➤ Blend the soup mixture into a blender. Serve and enjoy!

NUTRITION INFORMATION: Calories 545 Fats 50g Carbohydrates 10g Proteins 15g

38. KETO BUFFALO DRUMSTICKS WITH CHILI AIOLI AND GARLIC

Servings: 4   **Cook Time: 40 Min**   **Prep Time: 10 Min**

INGREDIENTS:

- ✓ 2 pounds (907g) chicken drumsticks or chicken wings
- ✓ 1/3 cup mayonnaise, keto-friendly
- ✓ 1 tbsp. smoked paprika powder or smoked chili powder
- ✓ 1 garlic clove, minced
- ✓ 2 tbsps. olive oil, and more for greasing the baking dish
- ✓ 2 tbsps. white wine vinegar
- ✓ 1 tsp. salt
- ✓ 1 tsp. paprika powder
- ✓ 1 tbsp. tabasco

DIRECTIONS:

- ➢ Now, preheat the oven to 450°F (235°C).
- ➢ Make the chili aioli: Combine the mayo, smoked paprika powder, garlic clove, olive oil white wine
- ➢ Add vinegar, salt, paprika powder and tabasco for the marinade in a small bowl,
- ➢ Put the drumsticks in a plastic bag, and pour the chili aioli into the plastic bag
- ➢ Shake the bag thoroughly and let marinate for 10 minutes at room temperature.
- ➢ Coat a baking dish with olive oil. Place the drumsticks in the baking dish
- ➢ Let bake in the preheated oven for 30 to 40 minutes or until they are done and have turned a nice color.
- ➢ Remove the chicken wings from the oven and serve warm.

NUTRITION INFORMATION: Calories: 570 Fat: 43.0g Carbs: 3.0g Protein: 43.0g

39. JERK PORK

Servings: 6   **Cook Time: 20 Min**   **Prep Time: 15 Min**

INGREDIENTS:

- ✓ 1/8 tsp cayenne pepper
- ✓ 1/4 tsp. salt
- ✓ 1/4 tsp. freshly ground black pepper
- ✓ 1/2 tbsp. dried thyme
- ✓ 1/2 tbsp. garlic powder
- ✓ 1/2 tbsp. ground allspice
- ✓ 1 tsp. ground cinnamon
- ✓ 1 tbsp. granulated erythritol
- ✓ 1 (1-pound/454-g) pork tenderloin, cut into 1-inch rounds
- ✓ 1/4 cup extra-virgin olive oil
- ✓ 2 tbsps. chopped fresh cilantro, for garnish
- ✓ 1/2 cup sour cream

DIRECTIONS:

- ➢ Combine the ingredients for the seasoning in a bowl. Stir to mix well.
- ➢ Put the pork rounds in the bowl of seasoning mixture. Toss to coat well.
- ➢ Pour the olive oil into a nonstick skillet, and heat over medium-high heat.
- ➢ Arrange the pork in the singer layer in the skillet and fry for 20 minutes
- ➢ (Or until an instant-read thermometer inserted in the center of the pork registers at least 145°F (63°C))
- ➢ Flip the pork rounds halfway through the cooking time. You may need to work in batches to avoid overcrowding.
- ➢ Transfer the pork rounds onto a large platter, and top with cilantro and sour cream, then serve warm.

NUTRITION INFORMATION: Calories: 289 Fat: 23.2g Carbs: 2.8g Protein: 17.2g

40. KETO CREAM CHEESE WITH WRAPS AND SALMON

Servings: 2   **Cook Time: 10 Min**   **Prep Time: 5 Min**

INGREDIENTS:

- ✓ 3 oz. of cream cheese
- ✓ 1 tbsp. of dill or other fresh herbs
- ✓ 1 oz. of smoked salmon
- ✓ 1 egg
- ✓ ½ oz. of butter
- ✓ Pinch of cayenne pepper
- ✓ Pepper and salt.

DIRECTIONS:

- ➤ Beat the egg well in a bowl. With 1 egg, you can make two thin wraps in a small frying pan.
- ➤ Melt the butter over medium heat in a small frying pan.
- ➤ Once the butter has melted, add half of the beaten egg to the pan.
- ➤ Move the pan back and forth so that the entire bottom is covered with a very thin layer of egg. Turn down the heat!
- ➤ Carefully loosen the egg on the edges with a silicone spatula
- ➤ Turn the wafer-thin omelets as soon as the egg is no longer dripping (about 45 seconds to 1 minute).
- ➤ You can do this by sliding it onto a lid or plate and then sliding it back into the pan.
- ➤ Let the other side be cooked for about 30 seconds and then remove from the pan.
- ➤ The omelets must be nice and light yellow. Repeat for the rest of the beaten egg.
- ➤ Once the omelets are ready, let them cool on a cutting board or plate and make the filling.
- ➤ Cut the dill into small pieces and put in a bowl
- ➤ Add the cream cheese, the salmon cut into small pieces, and mix together. Add a tiny bit of cayenne pepper and mix well. Taste immediately and then season with salt and pepper.
- ➤ Spread a layer on the wrap and roll it up. Cut the wrap in half and keep in the fridge until you are ready to eat it.

NUTRITION INFORMATION: Calories: 237 kcal Carbs: 14.7 g Protein: 15 g Fat: 5 g.

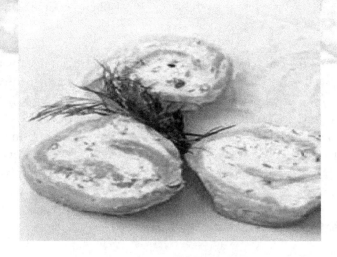

41. GRAVY BACON AND TURKEY

Servings: 14 **Cook Time: 3 H** **Prep Time: 15 Min**

INGREDIENTS:

- ✓ 12 pounds (5.4 kg) turkey
- ✓ Sea salt and fresh ground black pepper to taste
- ✓ 1-pound (454 g) cherry tomatoes
- ✓ 1 cup red onions, diced
- ✓ 2 garlic cloves, minced
- ✓ 1 large celery stalk, diced
- ✓ 4 tsp fresh thyme, four small sprigs
- ✓ 8 ounces (227 g) bacon (10 slices, diced)
- ✓ 8 tbsp butter
- ✓ 2 lemon, the juice

DIRECTIONS:

- ➤ Start by preheating the oven to 350°F.
- ➤ Remove the neck and giblets from the turkey, pat the turkey dry with paper towels and season both inside and outside of the turkey with salt and pepper. Insert cherry tomatoes, onions, celery, garlic, and thyme into the turkey
- ➤ cavity.
- ➤ Tie the legs together with kitchen twine and put the turkey on a large roasting pan, tuck its wings under the body.
- ➤ Cook the bacon in a large skillet over medium heat until crisp, for 7 to 8 minutes
- ➤ Transfer to paper towels to drain, reserving the drippings in the skillet.
- ➤ Add the ghee or butter to the skillet with the drippings and stir until melted, then pour into a bowl and stir in the lemon juice
- ➤ Rub mixture all over the turkey.
- ➤ Place into the oven for 30 minutes. After every 30 minutes, baste the turkey with the drippings
- ➤ Roast for about 3 hours or until a thermometer inserted into the thigh registers 165°F.
- ➤ Remove from oven onto a serving tray to rest for at least 25 minutes before serving.
- ➤ Meanwhile, pour the drippings into a saucepan. Then add the reserved bacon for a tasty gravy.
- ➤ Serve and enjoy!

NUTRITION INFORMATION: Calories 693 Fats 35.0g Carbohydrates 3.7g Fibers 0.7g Proteins 86.7g

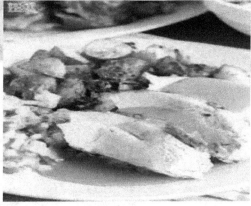

42. BELL PEPPER AND HOT PORK IN LETTUCE

Servings: 4   **Cook Time: 20 Min**   **Prep Time: 15 Min**

INGREDIENTS:
SAUCE:
- ✓ 1 tbsp. fish sauce
- ✓ 1 tbsp. rice vinegar
- ✓ 1 tbsp. almond flour

PORK FILLING:
- ✓ 2 tbsps. sesame oil, divided
- ✓ 1 pound (454 g) ground pork
- ✓ 1 tsp. fresh ginger, peeled and grated
- ✓ 1 tsp. garlic, minced

- ✓ 1 tsp. coconut aminos
- ✓ 1 tbsp. granulated erythritol
- ✓ 2 tbsps. coconut oil

- ✓ 1 red bell pepper, deseeded and thinly sliced
- ✓ 1 scallion, white and green parts, thinly sliced
- ✓ 8 large romaine or Boston lettuce leaves

DIRECTIONS:
- ➤ Make the sauce: Combine the ingredients for the sauce in a bowl. Set aside until ready to use.
- ➤ Make the pork filling: In a nonstick skillet, warm a tbsp. sesame oil over medium-high heat.
- ➤ Add the sauté the ground pork for 8 minutes or until lightly browned, then pour the sauce over
- ➤ Keep cooking for 4 minutes more or until the sauce has lightly thickened.
- ➤ Transfer the pork onto a platter and set aside until ready to use.

- ➤ Clean the skillet with paper towels, then warm the remaining sesame oil over medium-high heat.
- ➤ Add and sauté the ginger and garlic for 3 minutes or until fragrant.
- ➤ Add and sauté the sliced bell pepper and scallion for an additional 5 minutes or until fork-tender.
- ➤ Lower the heat, and move the pork back to the skillet. Stir to combine well.
- ➤ Divide and arrange the pork filling over four lettuce leaves and serve hot.

NUTRITION INFORMATION: Calories: 385 Fat: 31.1g Carbs: 5.8g Protein: 20.1g

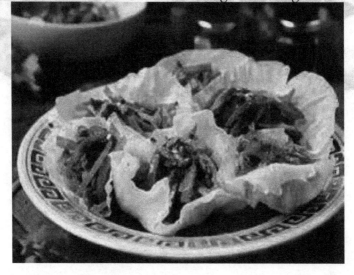

43. KETO-FRIENDLY SKILLET PEPPERONI PIZZA

Servings: 4   Cook Time: 6 Min   Prep Time: 10 Min

INGREDIENTS:

FOR THE CRUST:
- ✓ ½ cup almond flour
- ✓ ½ tsp baking powder

TOPPINGS:
- ✓ 3 tbsp unsweetened tomato sauce
- ✓ ½ cup shredded cheddar cheese

- ✓ 8 large egg whites, whisked into stiff peaks
- ✓ Salt and pepper to taste

- ✓ ½ cup pepperoni

DIRECTIONS:

- ➢ Gently incorporate the almond flour into the egg whites. Ensure that no lumps remain.
- ➢ Stir in the remaining crust ingredients.
- ➢ Heat a nonstick skillet over medium heat. Spray with nonstick spray. Pour the batter into the heated skillet to cover the bottom of the skillet.
- ➢ Cover the skillet with a lid

- ➢ Cook the pizza crust to cook for about 4 minutes or until bubbles that appear on the top.
- ➢ Flip the dough and add the toppings, starting with the tomato sauce and ending with the pepperoni
- ➢ Cook the pizza for 2 more minutes.
- ➢ Allow the pizza to cool slightly before serving. Enjoy!

NUTRITION INFORMATION: Calories 175 Carbohydrates 1.9g Fats 12g Proteins 14.3g

44. SESAME PORK WITH GREEN BEANS

Servings: 2   Cook Time: 10 Min   Prep Time: 5 Min

INGREDIENTS:

- ✓ 2 boneless pork chops
- ✓ Pink Himalayan salt
- ✓ Freshly ground black pepper
- ✓ 2 tbsp. toasted sesame oil, divided

- ✓ 2 tbsp. soy sauce
- ✓ 1 tsp. Sriracha sauce
- ✓ 1 cup fresh green beans.

DIRECTIONS:

- ➢ On a cutting board, pat the pork chops dry with a paper towel. Slice the chops into strips and season with pink Himalayan salt and pepper.
- ➢ In a large skillet over medium heat, heat one tablespoon of sesame oil. Add the pork strips and cook them for 7 minutes, stirring occasionally.

- ➢ In a small bowl, mix the remaining one tablespoon of sesame oil, the soy
- ➢ sauce, and the Sriracha sauce. Pour into the skillet with the pork.
- ➢ Add the green beans to the skillet, reduce the heat to medium-low, and simmer for 3 to 5 minutes.
- ➢ Divide the pork, green beans, and sauce between two wide, shallow bowls and serve.

NUTRITION INFORMATION: Calories: 387 kcal Fat: 15.1 g Carbs: 4.1 g Fiber: 10 g Protein: 18.1 g

45. PECAN PATTIES AND BACON, BEEF

Servings: 8 **Cook Time: 15 Min** **Prep Time: 10 Min**

INGREDIENTS:

- ✓ 1/4 cup chopped onion
- ✓ 1/4 cup ground pecans
- ✓ 1 large egg
- ✓ 8 ounces (227 g) bacon, chopped
- ✓ 1 pound (454 g) grass-fed ground beef
- ✓ Salt & freshly ground black pepper, to taste
- ✓ 1 tbsp. extra-virgin olive oil

DIRECTIONS:

- ➤ Now, preheat the oven to 450°F (235°C). Line a baking sheet with parchment paper.
- ➤ Whisk the ingredients, except for the olive oil, in a bowl.
- ➤ Grease your hands with olive oil, and shape the mixture into 8 patties with your hands.
- ➤ Arrange patties on a baking sheet and bake in the preheated oven for 20 min or until a meat thermometer inserted in the center of the patties reads at least 165°F (74°C)
- ➤ Flip patties halfway through cooking time.
- ➤ Remove the cooked patties from the oven and serve warm.

TIP: You can serve the patties with homemade sauces or store-bought burger toppings for more and different flavors.

NUTRITION INFORMATION: Calories: 318 Fat: 27.2g Carbs: 1.1g Protein: 18.1g

SNACKS RECIPES

46. SWISS CHEESE CRUNCHY NACHOS

Servings: 2   **Cook Time: 15 Min**   **Prep Time: 15 Min**

INGREDIENTS:
- ✓ ½ cup Swiss cheese
- ✓ ½ cup cheddar cheese
- ✓ 1/8 cup cooked bacon

DIRECTIONS:
- ➤ Heat-up the oven to 300°F.
- ➤ Spread the Swiss cheese on the greaseproof paper
- ➤ Sprinkle it with bacon and top it with the cheddar cheese.
- ➤ Bake for 10 minutes. Cool and cut into triangle strips
- ➤ Broil for 2 or 3 minutes. Serve and enjoy!

NUTRITION INFORMATION: Calories 280 Fats 21.8g Proteins 18.6g Carbohydrates 2.44g

47. BAKED CHORIZO

Servings: 6   **Cook Time: 30 Min**   **Prep Time: 10 Min**

INGREDIENTS:
- ✓ 7 oz. Spanish chorizo, sliced
- ✓ 1/4 cup chopped parsley

DIRECTIONS:
- ➤ Now, preheat the oven to 325 F
- ➤ Line a baking dish with waxed paper
- ➤ Bake the chorizo for minutes until crispy
- ➤ Remove from the oven and let cool.
- ➤ Arrange on a servings platter. Top each slice and parsley.

NUTRITION INFORMATION: Calories: 172 Carbs: 0.2g Fat: 13g Protein: 5g

48. HOMEMADE THIN MINTS

Servings: 20   **Cook Time: 60 Min**   **Prep Time: 15 Min**

INGREDIENTS:
- ✓ 1 egg
- ✓ 1 ¾ cups almond flour
- ✓ ⅓ cup cocoa powder
- ✓ ⅓ cup swerve sweetener
- ✓ 2 tbsp butter melted
- ✓ 1 tsp baking powder
- ✓ ½ tsp vanilla extract
- ✓ ¼ tsp salt
- ✓ 1 tbsp coconut oil
- ✓ 7 oz sugar-free dark chocolate
- ✓ 1 tsp peppermint extract

DIRECTIONS:
- ➤ Heat-up the oven to 300°F.
- ➤ Mix the cacao powder, sweetener, almond flour, salt and baking powder
- ➤ Then put the beaten egg, vanilla extract and butter.
- ➤ Knead the dough and roll it on the parchment paper. Cut into a cookie
- ➤ Bake the cookies for 20-30 minutes.
- ➤ For the coating, dissolve the oil and chocolate
- ➤ Stir in the peppermint extract
- ➤ Dip the cookie in the coating, chill, and serve. Enjoy!

NUTRITION INFORMATION: Calories 116 Fats 10.41g Carbohydrates 6.99g Proteins 8g

49. GOLDEN CRISPS

Servings: 4   **Cook Time: 10 Min**   **Prep Time: 10 Min**

INGREDIENTS:
- ✓ 1/3 tsp. dried oregano
- ✓ 1/3 tsp. dried rosemary
- ✓ 1/2 tsp. garlic powder
- ✓ 1/3 tsp. dried basil

DIRECTIONS:
- ➤ Now, preheat the oven to 390°F.
- ➤ In a small bowl mix the dried oregano, rosemary, basil, and garlic powder. Set aside.
- ➤ Line a large baking dish with parchment paper
- ➤ Sprinkle with the dry seasonings mixture and bake for 6-7 minutes.
- ➤ Let cool for a few minutes and enjoy.

NUTRITION INFORMATION: Calories: 296 Fat: 22.7g Carbs: 1.8g Protein: 22g

50. MOZZARELLA CHEESE POCKETS

Servings: 8   **Cook Time: 25 Min**   **Prep Time: 15 Min**

INGREDIENTS:
- ✓ 1 egg
- ✓ 8 mozzarella cheese sticks
- ✓ 1 ¾ cup mozzarella cheese
- ✓ ¾ cup almond flour
- ✓ 1 oz cream cheese
- ✓ ½ cup crushed pork rinds

DIRECTIONS:
- ➤ Grate the mozzarella cheese.
- ➤ Mix the almond flour, mozzarella, and cream cheese. Microwave for 30 seconds.
- ➤ Put in the egg and mix to form a dough.
- ➤ Put the dough in between two baking papers and roll it into a semi- rectangular shape.
- ➤ Cut them into smaller rectangle pieces and wrap them around the cheese sticks.
- ➤ Roll the stick onto crushed pork rinds.
- ➤ Bake about 20-25 minutes at 400°F. Serve and enjoy!

NUTRITION INFORMATION: Calories 272 Fats 22g Carbohydrates 2.4g Proteins 17g

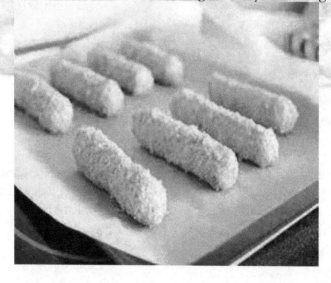

51. CRUNCHY RUTABAGA PUFFS

Servings: 4   Cook Time: 35 Min   Prep Time: 10 Min

INGREDIENTS:

- ✓ 1 rutabaga, peeled and diced
- ✓ 2 tbsp. melted butter
- ✓ 1/4 cup ground pork rinds
- ✓ Pinch of salt and black pepper

DIRECTIONS:

- ➤ Now, preheat the oven to 400 F and spread rutabaga on a baking sheet. Season with salt, pepper, and drizzle with butter.
- ➤ Bake until tender, minutes. Transfer to a bowl. Allow cooling. Using a fork, mash and mix the ingredients.
- ➤ Pour the pork rinds onto a plate. Mold 1-inch balls out of the rutabaga mixture and roll properly in the rinds while pressing gently to stick
- ➤ Place on the same baking sheet and bake for 10 minutes until golden.

NUTRITION INFORMATION: Calories: 129 Carbs: 5.9g Fat: 8g Protein: 3g

52. NO-BAKE COCONUT COOKIES

Servings: 8   Cook Time: 10 Min   Prep Time: 15 Min

INGREDIENTS:

- ✓ 3 cups unsweetened shredded coconut
- ✓ ½ cup sweetener
- ✓ 3/8 cup coconut oil
- ✓ 3/8 tsp salt
- ✓ 2 tsp vanilla

TOPPING:

- ✓ Coconut shreds

DIRECTIONS:

- ➤ Process all the fixing in a food processor
- ➤ Form into shape
- ➤ Put the topping. Chill and serve. Enjoy!

NUTRITION INFORMATION: Calories 329 Carbohydrates 4.1g Proteins 2.1g Fats 30g

53. HERBED COCONUT FLOUR BREAD

Servings: 2   Cook Time: 3 Min   Prep Time: 10 Min

INGREDIENTS:

- ✓ 4 tbsp. coconut flour
- ✓ 1/2 tsp. baking powder
- ✓ 1/2 tsp. dried thyme
- ✓ 2 tbsp. whipping cream
- ✓ 2 eggs

SEASONING:

- ✓ 1/2 tsp. oregano
- ✓ 2 tbsp. avocado oil

DIRECTIONS:

- ➤ Take a medium bowl, place all the ingredients in it and then whisk until incorporated and smooth batter comes together.
- ➤ Distribute the mixture evenly between two mugs and then microwave for a minute and 30 seconds until cooked.
- ➤ When done, take out bread from the mugs, cut it into slices, and then serve.

NUTRITION INFORMATION: Calories: 309 Fats: 26.1 g Protein: 9.3 g Carb: 4.3 g

54. KETO BEEF AND SAUSAGE BALLS

Servings: 3   **Cook Time: 20 Min**   **Prep Time: 15 Min**

INGREDIENTS:

MEATBALLS:
- ✓ 2 pounds ground beef
- ✓ 2 pounds ground sausage
- ✓ 2 eggs
- ✓ ½ cup keto mayo
- ✓ ⅓ cup ground pork rinds

SAUCE:
- ✓ 3 diced onions
- ✓ 2 pounds mushrooms
- ✓ 5 cloves garlic
- ✓ 3 cups beef broth
- ✓ 1 cup sour cream

- ✓ ½ cup Parmesan cheese
- ✓ Salt
- ✓ Pepper
- ✓ 2 tbsp butter
- ✓ 3tbsp oil

- ✓ 2 tbsp mustard
- ✓ Worcestershire sauce
- ✓ Salt
- ✓ Pepper Parsley
- ✓ 1 tbsp Arrowroot powder

DIRECTIONS:

- ➤ Put meat, egg, and onions in a bowl, mix.
- ➤ Put beef, Parmesan, egg, mayonnaise, sausage, pork rind in a bowl. Add salt and pepper. Warm-up oil in a skillet.
- ➤ Mold the beef mixture into balls, fry for 7-10 minutes. Put aside.
- ➤ Fry the diced onions, then the garlic and mushrooms, cook for 3 minutes

- ➤ Then, add the broth. Mix in mustard, sour cream, and Worcestershire sauce
- ➤ Boil for two minutes, then adds in the meatballs
- ➤ Add salt and pepper, simmer. Serve and enjoy!

NUTRITION INFORMATION: Calories 592 Fats 53.9g Carbohydrates 1.3g Proteins 25.4g

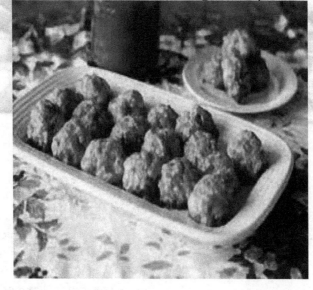

55. MINTY ZUCCHINIS

Servings: 4   **Cook Time: 15 Min**   **Prep Time: 10 Min**

INGREDIENTS:

- ✓ 1 pound zucchinis, sliced
- ✓ 1 tbsp. olive oil
- ✓ 2 garlic cloves, minced
- ✓ 1 tbsp. mint, chopped
- ✓ Pinch of salt and black pepper
- ✓ 1/4 cup veggie stock

DIRECTIONS:

- ➢ Heat up a pan with the oil over medium-high heat
- ➢ Add the garlic and sauté for 2 minutes.
- ➢ Then the zucchinis and the other ingredients
- ➢ Toss and cook everything for 10 minutes more, divide between plates and serve as a side dish.

NUTRITION INFORMATION: Calories: 70 Fat: 1g Carbs: 0.4g Protein: 6g

56. CHEESY MUSHROOM SLICES

Servings: 8   **Cook Time: 15 Min**   **Prep Time: 10 Min**

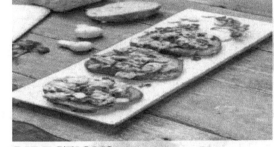

INGREDIENTS:

- ✓ 2 c. mushrooms
- ✓ 2 eggs
- ✓ ¾ c. almond flour
- ✓ ½ c. cheddar cheese
- ✓ 2 tbsp butter
- ✓ ½ tsp pepper
- ✓ ¼ tsp salt

DIRECTIONS:

- ➢ Process chopped mushrooms in a food processor then add eggs, almond flour and cheddar cheese.
- ➢ Put salt and pepper then pour melted butter into the food processor
- ➢ Transfer: Warm-up an Air Fryer to 375°F.
- ➢ Put the loaf on the air fryer's rack then cook within 15 minutes
- ➢ Slice and serve. Enjoy!

NUTRITION INFORMATION: Calories 365 - Fats 34.6g - Proteins 10.4g - Carbohydrates 4.4g

57. CRISPY CHORIZO WITH CHEESY TOPPING

Servings: 6   **Cook Time: 30 Min**   **Prep Time: 10 Min**

INGREDIENTS:

- ✓ 7 ounces Spanish chorizo, sliced 1/4 cup chopped parsley

DIRECTIONS:

- ➢ Preheat the oven to 325°F.
- ➢ Line a baking dish with waxed paper. Bake chorizo for minutes until crispy
- ➢ Remove and let cool.
- ➢ Arrange on a serving platter.
- ➢ Serve sprinkled with parsley.

NUTRITION INFORMATION: Calories: 172 Fat: 13g Carbs: 0g Protein: 5g

58. *ASPARAGUS FRIES*

Servings: 4   Cook Time: 10 Min   Prep Time: 10 Min

INGREDIENTS:

- ✓ 10 organic asparagus spears
- ✓ 1 tbsp organic roasted red pepper
- ✓ ¼ cup almond flour
- ✓ ½ tsp garlic powder
- ✓ ½ tsp smoked paprika
- ✓ 2 tbsp parsley
- ✓ ½ cup Parmesan cheese
- ✓ 2 organic eggs
- ✓ 3 tbsp keto mayo

DIRECTIONS:

- ➢ Warm-up oven to 425°F.
- ➢ Process cheese in a food processor, add garlic and parsley and pulse for 1 minute.
- ➢ Add almond flour, pulse for 30 seconds, transfer and put paprika
- ➢ Whisk eggs into a shallow dish.
- ➢ Dip asparagus spears into the egg batter, then coat with Parmesan mixture
- ➢ Place it on a baking sheet. Bake in the oven within 10 minutes.
- ➢ Put the mayonnaise in a bowl, add red pepper and whisk
- ➢ Then chill. Serve with prepared dip. Enjoy!

NUTRITION INFORMATION: Calories 453 Fats 33.4g Proteins 19.1g Carbohydrates 5.5g

59. *BUTTERNUT SQUASH ROAST & CRISPY PANCETTA*

Servings: 4   Cook Time: 30 Min   Prep Time: 10 Min

INGREDIENTS:

- ✓ 2 butternut squash, cubed
- ✓ 1 tsp. turmeric powder
- ✓ 1/2 tsp. garlic powder
- ✓ 8 pancetta slices, chopped
- ✓ 2 tbsp. olive oil
- ✓ 1 tbsp. chopped cilantro
- ✓ Pinch of salt and black pepper

DIRECTIONS:

- ➢ Preheat the oven to 425 F. In a bowl
- ➢ Add butternut squash, salt, pepper, turmeric, garlic powder, pancetta, and olive oil.
- ➢ Toss until well-coated.
- ➢ Spread the mixture onto a greased baking sheet and roast for -15 minutes
- ➢ Transfer the veggies to a bowl and garnish with cilantro to serve.

NUTRITION INFORMATION: Calories: 148 Carbs: 6.4g Fat: 10g Protein: 6g

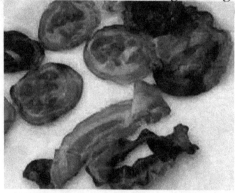

60. KALE CHIPS

Servings: 4   **Cook Time: 12 Min**   **Prep Time: 5 Min**

INGREDIENTS:
- ✓ 1 organic kale
- ✓ 1 tbsp seasoned salt
- ✓ 2 tbsp olive oil

DIRECTIONS:
- ➢ Warm up oven to 350°F.
- ➢ Put kale leaves into a large plastic bag and add oil
- ➢ Shake and then spread on a large baking sheet.
- ➢ Bake within 12 minutes. Serve with salt. Enjoy!

NUTRITION INFORMATION: Calories 163 Fats 10 g Proteins 2 g Carbohydrates 14 g

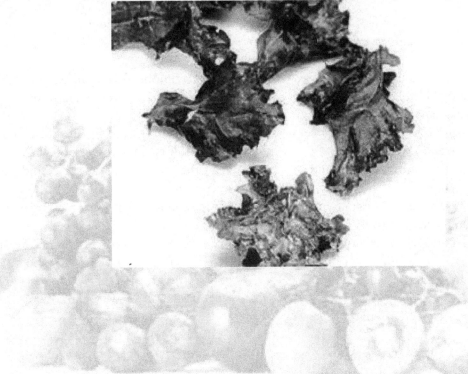

61. KETO FISH

Servings: 4   **Cook Time: 30 Min**   **Prep Time: 40 Min**

INGREDIENTS:

FOR THE TARTAR SAUCE:

- ✓ 4 tbsps. dill pickle relish
- ✓ 1 cup mayo
- ✓ 1/2 tbsp. curry powder

FOR THE FISH:

- ✓ 1 1/2 pounds white fish
- ✓ 1 cup almond flour
- ✓ 2 eggs
- ✓ 2 cups coconut oil, for frying

- ✓ 1 tbsp. olive oil
- ✓ 1 1/2 pounds rutabaga (peeled and cleaned)
- ✓ Salt and pepper, to taste

- ✓ 1 tsp. paprika powder
- ✓ 1/4 tsp. pepper
- ✓ 1/2 tsp. onion powder
- ✓ 1 tsp. salt

DIRECTIONS:

- ➢ Take a small bowl and mix mayonnaise, curry powder, and pickle relish thoroughly
- ➢ Refrigerate the tartar sauce until you finish the remaining dish.
- ➢ Now, preheat the oven to 400°F.
- ➢ Slice the peeled rutabaga into thin rods and brush them with oil.
- ➢ Line baking tray with parchment paper and spread the oil-coated rutabaga rods.
- ➢ Sprinkle the pepper and salt over the spread rutabaga.
- ➢ Bake for 30 minutes until the rods become golden brown.
- ➢ As the rutabaga gets cooked, prepare the fish.
- ➢ Crack eggs into small bowl and beat it well with a fork.
- ➢ Mix the almond flour, paprika powder, pepper, onion powder, and salt on a plate. Set aside.
- ➢ Dip the flour-coated fix into the beaten eggs and coat it again with the flour mix.
- ➢ Pour the oil in a shallow skillet and heat over high heat.
- ➢ If the rutabaga chips are ready by now, turn off the oven and let it sit for a while.
- ➢ Fry the flour-egg coated fish in the hot oil until the fish is completely cooked and turns golden brown.
- ➢ Repeat steps 11 and 14 with the remaining fish.
- ➢ Transfer the fried fish, baked rutabaga fries, and tartar into a serving bowl.
- ➢ Serve hot and enjoy!

NUTRITION INFORMATION: Calories: 463 Kcal Fat: 26.2 g Protein: 49.2 g Carb: 4 g

62. KORMA CURRY

Servings: 6   **Cook Time: 25 Min**   **Prep Time: 10 Min**

INGREDIENTS:

- ✓ 3-pound chicken breast, skinless, boneless
- ✓ 1 tsp. garam masala
- ✓ 1 tsp. curry powder
- ✓ 1 tbsp. apple cider vinegar
- ✓ ½ coconut cream
- ✓ 1 cup organic almond milk
- ✓ 1 tsp. ground coriander
- ✓ ¾ tsp. ground cardamom
- ✓ ½ tsp. ginger powder
- ✓ ¼ tsp. cayenne pepper
- ✓ ¾ tsp. ground cinnamon
- ✓ 1 tomato, diced
- ✓ 1 tsp. avocado oil
- ✓ ½ cup of water.

DIRECTIONS:

- ➢ Chop the chicken breast and put it in the saucepan. Add avocado oil and start to cook it over medium heat.
- ➢ Sprinkle the chicken with garam masala, curry powder, apple cider vinegar
- ➢ Then ground coriander, cardamom, ginger powder, cayenne pepper, ground cinnamon, and diced tomato
- ➢ Mix up the ingredients carefully.
- ➢ Cook them for 10 minutes.
- ➢ Add water, coconut cream, and almond milk. Sauté the meat for 10 minutes more.

NUTRITION INFORMATION: Calories: 440 kcal Fat: 32 g Fiber: 4 g Carbs: 28 g Protein: 8 g.

63. ZINGY LEMON FISH

Servings: 4   **Cook Time: 40 Min**   **Prep Time: 50 Min**

INGREDIENTS:

- ✓ 14 ounces fresh Gurnard fish fillets
- ✓ 2 tbsps. lemon juice
- ✓ 6 tbsps. butter
- ✓ 1/2 cup fine almond flour
- ✓ 2 teaspoons dried chives
- ✓ 1 tsp. garlic powder
- ✓ 2 teaspoons dried dill
- ✓ 2 teaspoons onion powder
- ✓ Salt and pepper to taste

DIRECTIONS:

- ➢ Add almond flour, dried herbs, salt, and spices on a large plate and stir until well combined. Spread it all over the plate evenly.
- ➢ Place a large pan over medium-high heat
- ➢ Add half the butter and half the lemon juice. When butter just melts, place fillets on the pan and cook for 3 minutes
- ➢ Move the fillets around the pan so that it absorbs the butter and lemon juice.
- ➢ Then remaining half butter and lemon juice. When butter melts, flip sides and cook the other side for 3 minutes.
- ➢ Serve fillets with any butter remaining in the pan.

NUTRITION INFORMATION: Calories: 406 Kcal Fat: 30.33 g Protein: 29 g Carb: 3.55 g

64. CHICKEN & CARROTS

Servings: 4　　　　　　　　Cook Time: 20 Min　　　　　　　　Prep Time: 15 Min

INGREDIENTS:

- ✓ 1 ½ lb. carrots, peeled and sliced
- ✓ 1 onion, sliced into quarters
- ✓ 1 head garlic, top sliced off
- ✓ 4 tbsp olive oil, divided
- ✓ Salt and pepper to taste
- ✓ 1 tbsp fresh rosemary, chopped
- ✓ 4 chicken thighs

DIRECTIONS:

- ➤ Preheat your oven to 425°F.
- ➤ Arrange the onion and carrots on a single layer on a baking pan.
- ➤ Place the garlic in the middle of the tray
- ➤ Drizzle half of the olive oil over the vegetables. Season with salt, pepper, and rosemary.
- ➤ Coat the chicken with the remaining oil. Season with salt and pepper.
- ➤ Bake in the oven for 20 minutes. Serve and enjoy!

NUTRITION INFORMATION: Calories 532 Fats 25.2g Carbohydrates 31.1g Fibers 5.8g Proteins 46.1g

65. CREAMY KETO FISH CASSEROLE

Servings: 4　　　　　　　　Cook Time: 50 Min　　　　　　　　Prep Time: 1 H

INGREDIENTS:

- ✓ 25 ounces of white fish (slice into bite-sized pieces)
- ✓ 15 ounces broccoli (small florets, include the step too)
- ✓ 3 ounces butter + extra
- ✓ 6 scallions (finely chopped)
- ✓ 1 1/4 cups heavy whipping cream
- ✓ 2 tbsps. small capers
- ✓ 1 tbsp. dried parsley
- ✓ 1 tbsp. Dijon mustard
- ✓ 1/4 tsp. black pepper (ground)
- ✓ 1 tsp. salt
- ✓ 2 tbsps. olive oil
- ✓ 5 ounces leafy greens (finely chopped), for garnishing

DIRECTIONS:

- ➤ Now, preheat the oven to 400°F
- ➤ Now, preheat the oven oil in a saucepan over medium-high heat.
- ➤ Fry the broccoli florets in the hot oil for 5 minutes until tender and golden.
- ➤ Transfer the fried florets to a small bowl and season it with salt and pepper
- ➤ Toss the contents to ensure all the florets get an equal amount of seasoning.
- ➤ Add the chopped scallions and capers to the same saucepan and fry for 2 minutes. Return the florets to the pan and mix well.
- ➤ Grease a baking tray with a little amount of butter and spread the fried veggies (broccoli, scallions, and capers) in the baking tray.
- ➤ Add the sliced fish to the tray and nestle it among the veggies.
- ➤ Mix the heavy cream, mustard, and parsley in a small bowl and pour this mixture over the fish-veggie mixture
- ➤ Top this with the remaining butter and spread gently over the contents using a spatula
- ➤ Transfer to a plate and garnish with chopped greens. Serve warm and enjoy!

NUTRITION INFORMATION: Calories: 822 Fat: 69 g Protein: 41 g Carb: 8 g

66. STICKY PORK RIBS

Servings: 8 **Cook Time: 2 H 30 Min** **Prep Time: 25 Min**

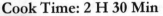

INGREDIENTS:
- ✓ ¼ cups granulated Erythritol
- ✓ 1 tbsp garlic powder
- ✓ 1 tbsp paprika
- ✓ ½ tsp red chili powder
- ✓ 4 pounds pork ribs, membrane removed
- ✓ Salt and ground black pepper, as required
- ✓ 1 ½ tsp liquid smoke
- ✓ 1 ½ cup sugar-free BBQ sauce

DIRECTIONS:
- ✓ Preheat your oven to 300°F.
- ✓ In a bowl, mix Erythritol, garlic powder, paprika and chili powder well. Season the ribs with pepper and salt. And then coat with the liquid smoke
- ✓ Rub the ribs evenly with Erythritol mixture.
- ✓ Arrange ribs onto the prepared baking sheet, meaty side down.
- ✓ Arrange two layers of foil on top of ribs and then roll and crimp edges tightly.
- ✓ Bake for about 2 – 2 ½ hours or until the desired doneness. Set the oven to broiler.
- ✓ With a sharp knife, cut the ribs into serving-sized portions and evenly coat with the barbecue sauce.
- ✓ Arrange the ribs onto a broiler pan, bony side up. Broil for about 1–2 minutes per side.
- ✓ Remove from the oven and serve hot. Enjoy!

NUTRITION INFORMATION: Calories 415 Fats 18.1g Fibers 12.5g Carbohydrates 3.1 g Proteins 18.5g

67. CREAMY ZOODLES

Servings: 4 **Cook Time: 10 Min** **Prep Time: 15 Min**

INGREDIENTS:
- ✓ 1¼ cups heavy whipping cream
- ✓ ¼ cup mayo
- ✓ Salt and ground black pepper, as required
- ✓ 30 oz. zucchini, spiralized with blade C
- ✓ 3 oz. Parmesan cheese, grated
- ✓ 2 tbsp. fresh mint leaves
- ✓ 2 tbsp. butter, melted.

DIRECTIONS:
- ➢ The heavy cream must be added to a pan then bring to a boil. Lower the heat to low and cook until reduced in half.
- ➢ Put in the pepper, mayo, and salt; cook until mixture is warm enough
- ➢ Add the zucchini noodles and gently stir to combine.
- ➢ Stir in the Parmesan cheese.
- ➢ Divide the zucchini noodles onto four serving plates and immediately drizzle with the melted butter.
- ➢ Serve immediately.

NUTRITION INFORMATION: Calories: 241 kcal Fat: 11.4 g Fiber: 7.5 g Carbs: 3.1 g Protein: 5.1 g.

68. KETO FISH CASSEROLE FRENCH MUSTARD, WITH MUSHROOMS

Servings: 6   **Cook Time: 50 Min**   **Prep Time: 1 H**

INGREDIENTS:

- ✓ 25 ounces of white fish
- ✓ 15 ounces mushrooms (cut into wedges)
- ✓ 20 ounces cauliflower (cut into florets)
- ✓ 2 cups heavy whipping cream
- ✓ 2 tbsps. Dijon mustard
- ✓ 3 ounces olive oil
- ✓ 2 tbsps. fresh parsley
- ✓ Salt & pepper, to taste

DIRECTIONS:

- ➤ Now, preheat the oven to 350°F
- ➤ Fry the mushroom for 5 minutes until tender and soft.
- ➤ Add the parsley, salt, and pepper to the mushrooms as you continue to mix well.
- ➤ Reduce the heat and add the mustard and heavy whipping cream to the mushroom.
- ➤ Allow it simmer for 10 minutes until the sauce thickens and reduces a bit.
- ➤ Season the fish slices with pepper and salt. Set aside.
- ➤ Spread the creamy mushroom over the top.
- ➤ Boil cauliflower florets in lightly salted water for 5 minutes and strain the water.
- ➤ Place the strained florets in a bowl and add the olive oil. Mash thoroughly with a fork until you get a coarse texture
- ➤ Season with salt and pepper. Mix well.

NUTRITION INFORMATION: Calories: 828 Fat: 71 g Protein: 39 g Carb: 8 g

69. CELERIAC GRATIN AND CREAMY PORK

Servings: 4   **Cook Time: 60 Min**   **Prep Time: 20 Min**

INGREDIENTS:

- ✓ ½ lb. celeriac, peeled and thinly sliced
- ✓ ⅓ cup almond milk
- ✓ ½ cup heavy cream
- ✓ ¼ tsp nutmeg powder
- ✓ Salt and black pepper to taste
- ✓ 1 tbsp olive oil
- ✓ 1 lb. ground pork
- ✓ ½ medium white onion, chopped
- ✓ 1 garlic clove, minced
- ✓ ½ tsp unsweetened tomato paste
- ✓ 3 tbsp butter for greasing
- ✓ 1 cup crumbled queso fresco cheese
- ✓ 1 tbsp chopped fresh parsley for garnish

DIRECTIONS:

- ➤ Let the oven preheat to 375°F.
- ➤ In a saucepan, add the celeriac, almond milk, heavy cream, nutmeg powder and salt.
- ➤ Cook until the celeriac softens. Drain afterward and set aside.
- ➤ Heat oil and cook the pork for 5 minutes or starting to brown.
- ➤ Season with salt and black pepper.
- ➤ Stir in the onion, garlic and cook for 5 minutes or until the onions soften. Add the tomato paste and continue cooking.
- ➤ Grease a baking dish and lay half of the celeriac on the bottom of the dish
- ➤ Spread the tomato-pork sauce on top and cover with the remaining celeriac
- ➤ Finish the topping with the queso fresco cheese.
- ➤ Let the gratin bake for about 45 minutes or until the cheese melts and is golden brown.
- ➤ Remove from the oven to cool for 5 to 10 minutes, garnish with the parsley
- ➤ Serve and enjoy!

NUTRITION INFORMATION: Calories 486 Fats 19.4g Fibers 10.3g Carbohydrates 8.5g Proteins 19.2g

70. KETO THAI FISH WITH CURRY AND COCONUT

Servings: 4   **Cook Time: 40 Min**   **Prep Time: 50 Min**

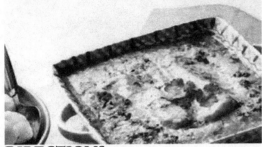

INGREDIENTS:

- ✓ 25 ounces salmon (slice into bite-sized pieces)
- ✓ 15 ounces cauliflower (bite-sized florets)
- ✓ 14 ounces coconut cream
- ✓ 1-ounce olive oil
- ✓ 4 tbsps. butter
- ✓ Salt and pepper, to taste

DIRECTIONS:

- ➤ Preheat the oven to 400°F
- ➤ Sprinkle salt and pepper over the salmon generously. Toss it once, if possible.
- ➤ Place the butter generously over all the salmon pieces and set aside.
- ➤ Pour this cream mixture over the fish in the baking tray.
- ➤ Meanwhile, boil the cauliflower florets in salted water for 5 minutes, strain and mash the florets coarsely. Set aside.
- ➤ Transfer the creamy fish to a plate and serve with mashed cauliflower. Enjoy!

NUTRITION INFORMATION: Calories: 880 Kcal Fat: 75 g Protein: 42 g Carb: 6 g

71. BAKED CRISPY CHICKEN

Servings: 12   **Cook Time: 40 Min**   **Prep Time: 10 Min**

INGREDIENTS:

- ✓ 4 oz pork rinds
- ✓ Salt and pepper to taste
- ✓ 1 tsp oregano
- ✓ 1 ½ tsp thyme
- ✓ 1 tsp smoked paprika
- ✓ ½ tsp garlic powder
- ✓ 12 chicken legs
- ✓ 2 oz mayo
- ✓ 1 egg
- ✓ 3 tbsp Dijon mustard

DIRECTIONS:

- ➤ Preheat your oven to 400°F.
- ➤ Grind pork rinds until they've turned into a powdery texture.
- ➤ Mix pork rinds with salt, pepper, oregano, thyme, paprika and garlic powder
- ➤ Spread mixture on a plate.
- ➤ In a bowl, mix the mayo, egg, and mustard.
- ➤ Dip each chicken leg first into the egg mixture then coat with the pork rind mixture.
- ➤ Bake in the oven for 40 minutes. Serve and enjoy!

NUTRITION INFORMATION: Calories 359 Fats 16.3g Carbohydrates 1.6g Fibers 0.3g Proteins 49g

72. CHEESY BACON SQUASH SPAGHETTI

Servings: 4   **Cook Time: 50 Min**   **Prep Time: 30 Min**

INGREDIENTS:

- ✓ 2 pounds spaghetti squash
- ✓ 2 pounds bacon
- ✓ ½ cup of butter
- ✓ 2 cups of shredded parmesan cheese
- ✓ Salt
- ✓ Black pepper.

DIRECTIONS:

Let the oven preheat to 375ºF.

- ➤ Trim or remove each stem of spaghetti squash
- ➤ Slice into rings no more than an inch wide, and take out the seeds.
- ➤ Lay the sliced rings down on the baking sheet, bake for 40-45 minutes.
- ➤ It is ready when the strands separate easily when a fork is used to scrape it. Let it cool.
- ➤ Cook sliced up bacon until crispy. Take out and let it cool.
- ➤ Take off the shell on each ring, separate each strand with a fork, and put them in a bowl.
- ➤ Heat the strands in a microwave to get them warm, then put in butter and stir around till the butter melts.
- ➤ Pour in parmesan cheese and bacon crumbles and add salt and pepper to your taste. Enjoy.

NUTRITION INFORMATION: Calories: 398 kcal Fat: 12.5 g Fiber: 9.4 g Carbs: 4.1 g Protein: 5.1 g.

73. ITALIAN CHICKEN

Servings: 4   **Cook Time: 15 Min**   **Prep Time: 10 Min**

INGREDIENTS:

- ✓ 2 tbsp olive oil
- ✓ 1 ½ lb. chicken breast meat, sliced thinly
- ✓ ½ cup chicken broth
- ✓ 1 cup heavy cream
- ✓ 1 tsp Italian seasoning
- ✓ ½ cup Parmesan cheese
- ✓ 1 tsp garlic powder
- ✓ 1 cup spinach, chopped
- ✓ ½ cup sun-dried tomatoes

DIRECTIONS:

- ➤ In a pan over medium heat add olive oil. Cook chicken for 4 to 5 minutes per side.
- ➤ Transfer chicken on a plate.
- ➤ Stir in the broth, cream, Italian seasoning, Parmesan cheese and garlic powder.
- ➤ Simmer until the sauce has thickened. Add the tomatoes and spinach.
- ➤ Cook until the spinach has wilted.
- ➤ Put the chicken back in the pan, stir well. Serve and enjoy!

NUTRITION INFORMATION: Calories 535 Fats 29.4g Carbohydrates 6.1g Fibers 1g Proteins 60.3g

74. CUCUMBER SAUCE WITH KETO SALMON TANDOORI

Servings: 4　　　　**Cook Time: 20 Min**　　　　**Prep Time: 15 Min**

INGREDIENTS:

- ✓ 25 ounces salmon (bite-sized pieces)
- ✓ 2 tbsps. coconut oil

FOR THE CUCUMBER SAUCE:

- ✓ 1/2 shredded cucumber (squeeze out the water completely)
- ✓ Juice of 1/2 lime

FOR THE CRISPY SALAD:

- ✓ 3 1/2 ounces lettuce (torn)
- ✓ 3 scallions (finely chopped)
- ✓ 2 avocados (cubed)

- ✓ 1 tbsp. tandoori seasoning

- ✓ 2 minced garlic cloves
- ✓ 1 1/4 cups sour cream or mayo
- ✓ 1/2 tsp. salt (optional)

- ✓ 1 yellow bell pepper (diced)
- ✓ Juice of 1 lime

DIRECTIONS:

- ➢ Preheat the oven to 350°F.
- ➢ Mix the tandoori seasoning with oil in a small bowl and coat the salmon pieces with this mixture.
- ➢ Bake for 20 minutes until soft and the salmon flakes with a fork.
- ➢ Take another bowl and place the shredded cucumber in it

- ➢ Add the mayo, minced garlic, and salt (if the mayo doesn't have salt) to the shredded cucumber.
- ➢ Mix the lettuce, scallions, avocados, and bell pepper in another bowl. Drizzle the contents with the lime juice.
- ➢ Transfer the veggie salad to a plate and place the baked salmon over it. Top the veggies and salmon with cucumber sauce.
- ➢ Serve immediately and enjoy!

NUTRITION INFORMATION: Calories: 847 Kcal Fat: 73 g Protein: 35 g Carb: 6 g

75. CREAMY MACKEREL

Servings: 4　　　　**Cook Time: 20 Min**　　　　**Prep Time: 10 Min**

INGREDIENTS:

- ✓ 2 shallots, minced
- ✓ 2 spring onions, chopped
- ✓ 2 tbsps. olive oil
- ✓ 4 mackerel fillets, skinless and cut into medium cubes

- ✓ 1 cup heavy cream
- ✓ 1 tsp. cumin, ground
- ✓ 1/2 tsp. oregano, dried
- ✓ A pinch of salt and black pepper
- ✓ 2 tbsps. chives, chopped

DIRECTIONS:

- ➢ Heat a pan with the oil over medium heat, add the spring onions and the shallots, stir and sauté for 5 minutes.
- ➢ Add the fish and cook it for 4 minutes.

- ➢ Add the rest of the ingredients, bring to a simmer, cook everything for 10 minutes more, divide between plates, and serve.

NUTRITION INFORMATION: Calories: 403 Fat: 33.9g Carbs: 2.7g Protein: 22g

76. SWEET & SOUR PORK

Servings: 4   **Cook Time: 15 Min**   **Prep Time: 15 Min**

INGREDIENTS:
- ✓ 1 lb pork chops
- ✓ Salt and pepper to taste
- ✓ ½ cup sesame seeds
- ✓ 2 tbsp peanut oil
- ✓ 2 tbsp soy sauce
- ✓ 3 tbsp apricot jam
- ✓ Chopped scallions

DIRECTIONS:
- ➢ Season pork chops with salt and pepper. Press sesame seeds on both sides of pork.
- ➢ Pour oil into a pan over medium heat
- ➢ Cook pork for 3 to 5 minutes per side. Transfer to a plate.
- ➢ In a bowl, mix soy sauce and apricot jam. Simmer for 3 minutes.
- ➢ Pour sauce over the pork and garnish with scallions before serving. Enjoy!

NUTRITION INFORMATION: Calories 414 Fats 27.5g Carbohydrates 12.9g Fibers 1.8g Proteins 29g

77. STUFFED PORTOBELLO MUSHROOMS

Servings: 4   **Cook Time: 10 Min**   **Prep Time: 10 Min**

INGREDIENTS:
- ✓ 2 portobello mushrooms
- ✓ 1 cup spinach, chopped, steamed
- ✓ 2 oz. artichoke hearts, drained, chopped
- ✓ 1 tbsp. coconut cream
- ✓ 1 tbsp. cream cheese
- ✓ 1 tsp. minced garlic
- ✓ 1 tbsp. fresh cilantro, chopped
- ✓ 3 oz. Cheddar cheese, grated
- ✓ ½ tsp. ground black pepper
- ✓ 2 tbsp. olive oil
- ✓ ½ tsp. salt.

DIRECTIONS:
- ➢ Sprinkle mushrooms with olive oil and place in the tray.
- ➢ Transfer the tray to the preheated to 360°F oven and broil them for 5 minutes.
- ➢ Meanwhile, blend artichoke hearts, coconut cream, cream cheese, minced garlic, and chopped cilantro.
- ➢ Add grated cheese to the mixture and sprinkle with ground black pepper and salt.
- ➢ Fill the broiled mushrooms with the cheese mixture and cook them for 5 minutes more. Serve the mushrooms only hot.

NUTRITION INFORMATION: Calories: 135.2 kcal Total Fat: 5.5 g Cholesterol: 16.4 mg Sodium: 698.1 mg Potassium: 275.3 mg Carbs: 8.4 g Protein: 14.8 g.

78. LIME MACKEREL

Servings: 4   **Cook Time: 30 Min**   **Prep Time: 10 Min**

INGREDIENTS:
- ✓ 4 mackerel fillets, boneless
- ✓ 2 tbsps. lime juice
- ✓ 2 tbsps. olive oil
- ✓ A pinch of salt and black pepper
- ✓ 1/2 tsp. sweet paprika

DIRECTIONS:
- ➢ Arrange the mackerel on a baking sheet lined with parchment paper
- ➢ Add the oil and the other ingredients, rub gently, introduce in the oven at 360°F and bake for 30 minutes.
- ➢ Divide the fish between plates and serve.

NUTRITION INFORMATION: Calories: 297 Fat: 22.7g Carbs: 2g Protein: 21.1g

79. BEEF SHANKS BRAISED IN RED WINE SAUCE

Servings: 5   **Cook Time: 3 H**   **Prep Time: 20 Min**

INGREDIENTS:
- ✓ 2 tbsp olive oil
- ✓ 2 pounds (907 g) beef shanks
- ✓ 2 cups dry red wine
- ✓ 3 cups beef stock
- ✓ 1 sprig of fresh rosemary
- ✓ 5 garlic cloves, finely chopped
- ✓ 1 onion, finely chopped
- ✓ Pepper and salt

DIRECTIONS:
- ➢ Heat olive oil.
- ➢ Put the beef shanks into the skillet and fry for 5 to 10 minutes until well browned.
- ➢ Slice the beef shanks halfway through. Set aside
- ➢ Pour red wine into the pot and let it simmer.
- ➢ Add the cooked beef shanks, dry red wine, beef stock, rosemary
- ➢ Then garlic, onion, salt and black pepper to the slow cooker. Stir to mix well.
- ➢ Slow cook with the lid on for 3 hrs. Serve and enjoy!

NUTRITION INFORMATION: Calories 341 - Fats 19.6g - Fibers 10 g - Carbohydrates 15.4g - Proteins 21.6g

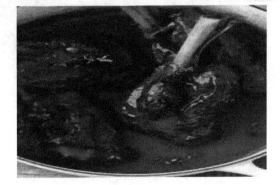

80. PESTO FLAVORED STEAK

Servings: 4   **Cook Time: 17 H**   **Prep Time: 15 Min**

INGREDIENTS:

- ✓ ¼ cup fresh oregano, chopped
- ✓ 1½ tbsp. garlic, minced
- ✓ 1 tbsp. fresh lemon peel, grated
- ✓ ½ tsp. red pepper flakes, crushed
- ✓ Salt and freshly ground black pepper, to taste
- ✓ 1 lb. (1-inch thick) grass-fed boneless beef top sirloin steak
- ✓ 1 cup pesto
- ✓ ¼ cup feta cheese, crumbled.

DIRECTIONS:

- ➢ Preheat the gas grill to medium heat. Lightly, grease the grill grate.
- ➢ In a bowl, add the oregano, garlic, lemon peel, red pepper flakes, salt, black pepper, and mix well.
- ➢ Rub the garlic mixture onto the steak evenly.
- ➢ Place the steak onto the grill and cook, covered for about 12-17 minutes, flipping occasionally.
- ➢ Remove from the grill and place the steak onto a cutting board for about 5 minutes.
- ➢ With a sharp knife, cut the steak into desired sized slices.
- ➢ Divide the steak slices and pesto onto serving plates and serve with the topping of the feta cheese.

NUTRITION INFORMATION: Calories: 226 kcal Carbs: 6.8 g Sugar: 0.7 g Fiber: 2.2 g Protein: 40.5 g Fat: 7.6 g Sodium: 579 mg.

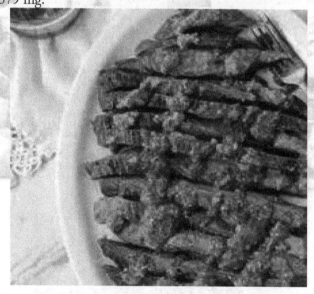

81. MOCHA MOUSSE

Servings: 4   **Cook Time: 0 Min**   **Prep Time: 2 H 35 Min**

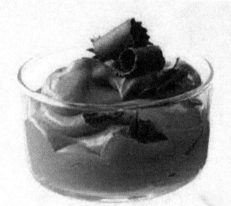

INGREDIENTS:

- ✓ 3 tbsps. sour cream, full-fat
- ✓ 2 tbsps. butter, softened
- ✓ 1 1/2 teaspoons vanilla extract, unsweetened
- ✓ 1/3 cup erythritol
- ✓ 1/4 cup cocoa powder, unsweetened
- ✓ 3 teaspoons instant coffee powder

FOR THE WHIPPED CREAM:

- ✓ 2/3 cup heavy whipping cream, full-fat
- ✓ 1 1/2 tsp. erythritol
- ✓ 1/2 tsp. vanilla extract, unsweetened

DIRECTIONS:

- ➢ Add sour cream and butter then beat until smooth.
- ➢ Now add erythritol, cocoa powder, coffee, and vanilla and blend until incorporated, set aside until required.
- ➢ Prepare whipping cream: For this, place whipping cream in a bowl and beat until soft peaks form.
- ➢ Beat in vanilla and erythritol until stiff peaks form, and fold until just mixed.
- ➢ Then add remaining whipping cream mixture and fold until evenly incorporated.
- ➢ Spoon the mousse into a freezer-proof bowl and place in the refrigerator for 2 1/2 hours until set.
- ➢ Serve straight away.

NUTRITION INFORMATION: Calories: 421.7 Fat: 42 g Protein: 6 g Carbs: 6.5 g

82. KETO SHAKE

Servings: 1   **Cook Time: 0 Min**   **Prep Time: 25 Min**

INGREDIENTS:

- ✓ ¾ cup almond milk
- ✓ ½ cup ice
- ✓ 2 tbsp almond butter
- ✓ 2 tbsp unsweetened cocoa powder
- ✓ 2 tbsp Swerve
- ✓ 1 tbsp chia seeds
- ✓ 2 tbsp hemp seeds
- ✓ ½ tbsp vanilla extract
- ✓ Salt to taste

DIRECTIONS:

- ➢ Blend all the ingredients in a food processor
- ➢ Chill in the refrigerator before serving. Enjoy!

NUTRITION INFORMATION: Calories 104 Carbohydrates 3.6g Proteins 2.9g Fats 9.5g Fibers 1.4g

83. KETO CHEESECAKES

Servings: 9   **Cook Time: 15 Min**   **Prep Time: 25 Min**

INGREDIENTS:

FOR THE CHEESECAKES:
- ✓ 1 tbsp butter
- ✓ 1 tbsp caramel syrup; sugar-free
- ✓ 3 tbsp coffee
- ✓ 8 ounces cream cheese

- ✓ ⅓ cup swerve
- ✓ 3 eggs

FOR THE FROSTING:
- ✓ 8 ounces mascarpone cheese; soft
- ✓ 3 tbsp caramel syrup; sugar-free

- ✓ 2 tbsp swerve
- ✓ 3 tbsp butter

DIRECTIONS:

➢ In the blender, mix cream cheese with eggs, 2 tbsp butter, coffee, 1 tbsp caramel syrup and ⅓ cup swerve and pulse very well.

➢ Spoon this into a cupcakes pan, introduce in the oven at 350°F and bake for 15 minutes.

➢ Set aside to cool down.

➢ Meanwhile, in a bowl, mix 3 tbsp butter with 3 tbsp caramel syrup, 2 tbsp swerve, and mascarpone cheese and blend well.

➢ Spoon this over cheesecakes and serve them. Enjoy!

NUTRITION INFORMATION: Calories 478.2 Fats 47.8g Carbohydrates 9.4g Proteins 9.2g

84. BAKED APPLES

Servings: 4   **Cook Time: 1 H**   **Prep Time: 10 Min**

INGREDIENTS:
- ✓ 3 tsp. or to taste Keto-friendly sweetener
- ✓ ¾ tsp. cinnamon

- ✓ ¼ cup chopped pecans
- ✓ 4 large granny Smith apples.

DIRECTIONS:

➢ Set the oven temperature at 375°F. Mix the sweetener with the cinnamon and pecans.

➢ Core the apple and add the prepared stuffing.

➢ Add enough water into the baking dish to cover the bottom of the apple

➢ Bake them for about 45 minutes to 1 hour.

NUTRITION INFORMATION: Calories: 175 kcal Carbs: 16 g Protein: 6.8 g Fats: 19.9 g.

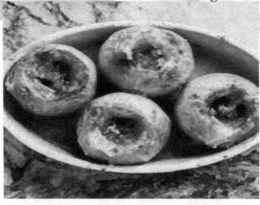

85. PUMPKIN PIE PUDDING

Servings: 4   **Cook Time: 20 Min**   **Prep Time: 4 H 25 Min**

INGREDIENTS:

- ✓ 2 eggs
- ✓ 1 cup heavy whipping cream, divided
- ✓ 3/4 cup erythritol sweetener
- ✓ 15 ounces pumpkin puree
- ✓ 1 tsp. pumpkin pie spice
- ✓ 1 tsp. vanilla extract, unsweetened
- ✓ 1 1/2 cup water

DIRECTIONS:

- ➤ Crack eggs in a bowl, add 1/2 cup cream, sweetener, pumpkin puree, pumpkin pie spice, and vanilla and whisk until blended.
- ➤ Take a 6 by 3-inch baking pan, grease it well with avocado oil, then pour in egg mixture, smooth the top and cover with aluminum foil.
- ➤ Switch on the instant pot, pour in water, insert a trivet stand and place baking pan on it.
- ➤ Shut the instant pot with its lid in the sealed position
- ➤ Then press the 'manual' button, press '+/-' to the set the cooking time to 20 minutes & cook at high-pressure setting
- ➤ When the pressure builds in the pot, the cooking timer will start.
- ➤ During the instant pot buzzes, press the 'keep warm' button, release pressure naturally for 10 min, and then do quick pressure release and open the lid.
- ➤ Take out the baking pan, uncover it, let cool for 15 minutes at room temperature, then transfer the pan into the refrigerator for 4 hours or until cooled.
- ➤ Top pie with remaining cream, then cut it into slices and serve

NUTRITION INFORMATION: Calories: 184 Fat: 16 g Protein: 3 g Carbs: 5 g

86. KETO BROWNIES

Servings: 12   **Cook Time: 20 Min**   **Prep Time: 30 Min**

INGREDIENTS:

- ✓ 6 ounces coconut oil; melted
- ✓ 4 ounces cream cheese
- ✓ 5 tbsp swerve
- ✓ 6 eggs
- ✓ 2 tsp vanilla
- ✓ 3 ounces of cocoa powder
- ✓ ½ tsp baking powder

DIRECTIONS:

- ➤ In a blender, mix eggs with coconut oil, cocoa powder, baking powder, vanilla, cream cheese and swerve and stir using a mixer.
- ➤ Pour this into a lined baking dish, introduce in the oven at 350°F and bake for 20 minutes.
- ➤ Slice into rectangle pieces when their cold. Serve and enjoy!

NUTRITION INFORMATION: Calories 183.7 Fats 16.6g Carbohydrates 4.9g Proteins 1.4g

87. AVOCADO & CHOCOLATE PUDDING

Servings: 2   **Cook Time: 10 Min**   **Prep Time: 20 Min**

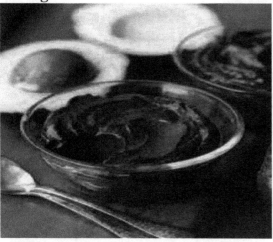

INGREDIENTS:
- ✓ 1 ripe medium avocado
- ✓ 1 tsp. natural sweetener
- ✓ 1/4 tsp. vanilla extract
- ✓ 4 tbsp. unsweetened cocoa powder
- ✓ 1 pinch pink salt

DIRECTIONS:
- ➤ Combine the avocado, sweetener, vanilla, cocoa powder, and salt into the blender or processor.
- ➤ Pulse until creamy smooth.
- ➤ Measure into fancy dessert dishes and chill for at least 1/2 hour.

NUTRITION INFORMATION: Calories: 281 Carbs: 2 g Protein: 8 g Fat: 27 g

88. RASPBERRY AND COCONUT

Servings: 12   **Cook Time: 5 Min**   **Prep Time: 15 Min**

INGREDIENTS:
- ✓ ¼ cup swerve
- ✓ ½ cup coconut oil
- ✓ ½ cup raspberries; dried
- ✓ ½ cup coconut; shredded
- ✓ ½ cup coconut butter

DIRECTIONS:
- ➤ In your food processor, blend dried berries very well
- ➤ Heat a pan with the butter over medium heat.
- ➤ Add oil, coconut and swerve; stir and cook for 5 minutes. Pour half of this into a lined baking pan and spread well. Add raspberry powder and spread.
- ➤ Top with the rest of the butter mix, spread, and keep in the fridge for a while
- ➤ Cut into pieces and serve. Enjoy!

NUTRITION INFORMATION: Calories 185 - Carbohydrates 45g - Fats 42g - Proteins 8g

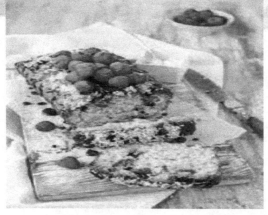

89. *CAKE PUDDING*

Servings: 4   **Cook Time: 5 Min**   **Prep Time: 5 Min**

INGREDIENTS:

- ✓ ½ heavy whipping cream
- ✓ 1 tsp. lemon juice
- ✓ ½ sour cream
- ✓ 20 drops liquid stevia
- ✓ 1 tsp. vanilla extract

DIRECTIONS:

- ➢ Whip the sour cream and whipping cream together with the mixer until soft peaks form
- ➢ Combine with the rest of the ingredients and whip until fluffy.

- ➢ Portion into four dishes to chill. Place a layer of the wrap over the dish and store in the fridge.
- ➢ When ready to eat, garnish with some berries if you like.
- ➢ Note: If you add berries, be sure to add the carbs.

NUTRITION INFORMATION: Calories: 356 Carbs: 5 g Protein: 5 g Fat: 36 g

90. *CHOCOLATE PUDDING DELIGHT*

Servings: 2   **Cook Time: 5 Min**   **Prep Time: 52 Min**

INGREDIENTS:

- ✓ ½ tsp stevia powder
- ✓ 2 tbsp cocoa powder
- ✓ 2 tbsp water
- ✓ 1 tbsp gelatin
- ✓ 1 cup of coconut milk
- ✓ 2 tbsp maple syrup

DIRECTIONS:

- ➢ Heat a pan with the coconut milk over medium heat
- ➢ Add stevia and cocoa powder and stir well.
- ➢ In a bowl, mix gelatin with water; stir well and add to the pan.

- ➢ Stir well, add maple syrup, whisk again, divide into ramekins and keep in the fridge for 45 minutes
- ➢ Serve cold and enjoy!

NUTRITION INFORMATION: Calories 221.2 - Fats 13.6g - Carbohydrates 22.7g - Proteins 3.4g

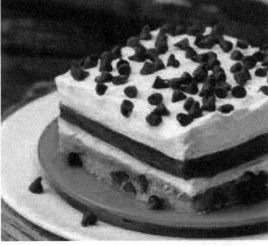

91. *CARROT ALMOND CAKE*

Servings: 8   **Cook Time: 15 Min**   **Prep Time: 45 Min**

INGREDIENTS:

- ✓ 3 eggs
- ✓ 1 ½ tsp. apple pie spice
- ✓ 1 cup almond flour
- ✓ 2/3 cup swerve
- ✓ 1 tsp. baking powder
- ✓ 1/4 cup coconut oil
- ✓ 1 cup shredded carrots
- ✓ 1/2 cup heavy whipping cream
- ✓ 1/2 cup chopped walnuts

DIRECTIONS:

- ➢ Grease cake pan. Combine all of the ingredients with the mixer until well mixed. Pour the mix into the pan and cover with a layer of foil.
- ➢ Pour two cups of water into the Instant Pot bowl along with the steamer rack.
- ➢ Arrange the pan on the trivet and set the pot using the cake button (40 min.).
- ➢ Natural-release the pressure for ten minutes. Then, quick-release the rest of the built-up steam pressure.
- ➢ Cool then start frosting or serve it plain.

NUTRITION INFORMATION: Calories: 268 Carbs: 4 g Fat: 25 g Protein: 6 g

92. *PEANUT BUTTER FUDGE*

Servings: 12   **Cook Time: 5 Min**   **Prep Time: 2 H 12 Min**

INGREDIENTS:

- ✓ 1 cup peanut butter; unsweetened
- ✓ 1 cup of coconut oil
- ✓ ¼ cup almond milk
- ✓ 2 tbsp vanilla stevia
- ✓ A pinch of salt

FOR THE TOPPING:

- ✓ 2 tbsp swerve
- ✓ ¼ cup cocoa powder
- ✓ 2 tbsp melted coconut oil

DIRECTIONS:

- ➢ In a heatproof bowl, mix peanut butter with 1 cup coconut oil; stir and heat up in your microwave until it melts.
- ➢ Add a pinch of salt, almond milk, and stevia; stir well everything and pour into a lined loaf pan.
- ➢ Keep in the fridge for 2 hours and then slice it.
- ➢ In a bowl, mix 2 tbsp melted coconut with cocoa powder and swerve and stir very well.
- ➢ Drizzle the sauce over your peanut butter fudge. Serve and enjoy!

NUTRITION INFORMATION: Calories 85 Carbohydrates 40g Fats 4.7g Proteins 0.5g

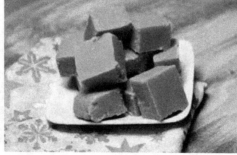

93. *CHOCOLATE LAVA CAKE*

Servings: 4   **Cook Time: 10 Min**   **Prep Time: 20 Min**

INGREDIENTS:

- ✓ ½ cup unsweetened cocoa powder
- ✓ ¼ cup melted butter
- ✓ 4 eggs
- ✓ ¼ tsp. sugar-free chocolate sauce
- ✓ ½ tsp. sea salt
- ✓ ½ tsp. ground cinnamon
- ✓ Pure vanilla extract
- ✓ ¼ cup Stevia
- ✓ Also Needed: Ice cube tray & 4 ramekins

DIRECTIONS:

- ➤ Pour one tbsp. of the chocolate sauce into four of the tray slots and freeze.
- ➤ Warm up the oven to 350°Fahrenheit. Lightly grease the ramekins with butter or a spritz of oil.
- ➤ Mix salt, cinnamon, cocoa powder, & stevia until combined. Whisk in the eggs – one at a time. Stir in the melted vanilla extract and butter.
- ➤ Fill each of the ramekins halfway & add one of the frozen chocolates. Cover the rest of the container with the cake batter.
- ➤ Bake 13-14 min. When they're set, place on a wire rack to cool for about five minutes. Remove and put on a serving dish.
- ➤ Enjoy by slicing its molten center.

NUTRITION INFORMATION: Calories: 189 Carbs: 3 g Protein: 8 g Fat: 17 g

94. *KETO FROSTY*

Servings: 4   **Cook Time: 0 Min**   **Prep Time: 45 Min**

INGREDIENTS:

- ✓ 1 ½ cups heavy whipping cream
- ✓ 2 tbsp unsweetened cocoa powder
- ✓ 3 tbsp Swerve
- ✓ 1 tsp pure vanilla extract
- ✓ Salt to taste

DIRECTIONS:

- ➤ In a bowl, combine all the ingredients.
- ➤ Use a hand mixer and beat until you see stiff peaks forming
- ➤ Place the mixture in a Ziploc bag.
- ➤ Freeze for 35 minutes.
- ➤ Serve in bowls or glasses. Enjoy!

NUTRITION INFORMATION: Calories 164 Fats 17g Carbohydrates 2.9g Fibers 0.8g Proteins 1.4g

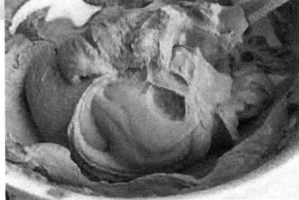

95. KETO FAT BOMBS

Servings: 10   **Cook Time: 0 Min**   **Prep Time: 30 Min**

INGREDIENTS:

- ✓ 8 tbsp butter
- ✓ ¼ cup Swerve
- ✓ ½ tsp vanilla extract
- ✓ Salt to taste
- ✓ 2 cups almond flour
- ✓ 2/3 cup chocolate chips

DIRECTIONS:

- ➢ In a bowl, beat the butter until fluffy. Stir in the sugar, salt and vanilla.
- ➢ Mix well.
- ➢ Add the almond flour. Fold in the chocolate chips.
- ➢ Cover the bowl with cling wrap and refrigerate for 20 minutes
- ➢ Create balls from the dough. Serve and enjoy!

NUTRITION INFORMATION: Calories 176 Carbohydrates 12.9g Fats 15.2g Proteins 2.2g Fibers 1g

96. GLAZED POUND CAKE

Servings: 16   **Cook Time: 1 H**   **Prep Time: 1 H**

INGREDIENTS:

- ✓ ½ tsp. salt
- ✓ 2 ½ cup almond flour
- ✓ ½ cup unsalted butter
- ✓ 1 ½ cup erythritol

THE GLAZE:

- ✓ ¼ cup powdered erythritol
- ✓ 3 tbsp. heavy whipping cream
- ✓ 8 unchilled eggs
- ✓ ½ tsp. lemon extract
- ✓ 1 ½ tsp. vanilla extract
- ✓ 1 ½ tsp. baking powder

- ✓ ½ tsp. vanilla extract

DIRECTIONS:

- ➢ Warm the oven to 350°Fahrenheit.
- ➢ Whisk together baking powder, almond flour, and salt
- ➢ Cream the erythritol, butter. Mix until smooth in a large mixing container.
- ➢ Whisk and add the eggs with the lemon and vanilla extract
- ➢ Blend with the rest of the ingredients using a hand mixer until smooth.
- ➢ Dump the batter into a loaf pan. Bake for one to two hours.
- ➢ Prepare a glaze. Mix in vanilla extract, powdered erythritol, and heavy whipping cream until smooth.
- ➢ You should let the cake cool completely before adding the glaze.

NUTRITION INFORMATION: Calories: 254 Carbs: 2.5 g Protein: 7.9 g Fat: 23.4 g

97. AVOCADO ICE POPS

Servings: 10   **Cook Time: 1 Min**   **Prep Time: 20 Min**

INGREDIENTS:

- ✓ 3 avocados
- ✓ ¼ cup lime juice
- ✓ 3 tbsp Swerve
- ✓ ¾ cup of coconut milk
- ✓ 1 tbsp coconut oil
- ✓ 1 cup keto-friendly chocolate

DIRECTIONS:

- ➤ Add all the ingredients except the oil and chocolate in a blender. Blend until smooth.
- ➤ Pour the mixture into the popsicle mold. Freeze overnight.
- ➤ In a bowl, mix oil and chocolate chips. Melt in the microwave. And then let cool.
- ➤ Dunk the avocado popsicles into the chocolate before serving. Enjoy!

NUTRITION INFORMATION: Calories 176 Carbohydrates 10.8g Proteins 1.6g Fats 17.4g Fibers 4.5g

98. LEMON CAKE

Servings: 8   **Cook Time: 2 H**   **Prep Time: 1 H 30 Min**

INGREDIENTS:

- ✓ ½ cup coconut flour
- ✓ 2 tsp. baking powder.
- ✓ 1 ½ cups almond flour
- ✓ 3 tbsp. Swerve (or) Pyure A-P.
- ✓ ½ tsp. Xanthan gum
- ✓ ½ cup whipping cream
- ✓ ½ cup melted butter
- ✓ 2 lemons zested & juiced
- ✓ 2 Eggs

INGREDIENTS FOR THE TOPPING:

- ✓ 3 tbsp. Pyure all-purpose/Swerve
- ✓ 2 tbsp. lemon juice
- ✓ ½ cup boiling water
- ✓ 2 tbsp. melted butter
- ✓ Suggested: 2-4-quart slow cooker

DIRECTIONS:

FOR THE CAKE:

- ➤ Mix the dry ingredients in a container.
- ➤ Whisk the egg with the lemon juice and zest, butter, and whipping cream.

FOR THE TOPPING:

- ➤ Mix all of the topping ingredients in a container and empty over the batter in the cooker.

- ➤ Whisk all of the ingredients and scoop out the dough into the prepared slow cooker.

- ➤ Place the lid on the cooker for two to three hours on the high setting.
- ➤ Serve warm with some fresh fruit or whipped cream.

NUTRITION INFORMATION: Calories: 350 Carbs: 5.2 g Protein: 7.6 g Fat: 33 g

99. CINNAMON STREUSEL EGG LOAF

Servings: 2   **Cook Time: 15 Min**   **Prep Time: 10 Min**

INGREDIENTS:

- ✓ 2 tbsp almond flour
- ✓ 1 tbsp butter, softened
- ✓ ½ tbsp grated butter, chilled
- ✓ 1 egg
- ✓ 1-ounce cream cheese
- ✓ ½ tsp cinnamon, divided
- ✓ 1 tbsp Erythritol sweetener, divided
- ✓ ¼ tsp vanilla extract, unsweetened

DIRECTIONS:

- ➢ Turn on the oven, then set it to 350°F and let it preheat.
- ➢ Meanwhile, crack the egg in a small bowl
- ➢ Add cream cheese, softened butter, ¼ tsp cinnamon, ½ tbsp sweetener, and vanilla and whisk until well combined.
- ➢ Divide the egg batter between two silicone muffins and then bake for 7 minutes.
- ➢ Meanwhile, prepare the streusel and for this, place flour in a small bowl, add remaining ingredients and stir until well mixed.
- ➢ When egg loaves have baked, sprinkle streusel on top and then continue baking for 7 minutes.
- ➢ When done, remove loaves from the cups, let them cool for 5 minutes and then Serve and enjoy!

NUTRITION INFORMATION: Calories 152 Carbohydrates 1.3g Fats 14.8g Proteins 4.1g Fibers 0.9g

100.   RASPBERRY FUDGE

Servings: 12   **Cook Time: 1 H**   **Prep Time: 1 H 15 Min**

INGREDIENTS:

- ✓ 1 cup butter
- ✓ ¼ cup white sugar substitute
- ✓ 6 tbsp. unsweetened cocoa powder
- ✓ 2 tbsp. heavy cream
- ✓ 2 tsp. vanilla extract
- ✓ 1 tsp. raspberry extract
- ✓ 1/3 cup chopped walnuts

DIRECTIONS:

- ➢ Put the butter in the mixing bowl with the mixer.
- ➢ When smooth, mix with the rest of the ingredients until well incorporated.
- ➢ Microwave using the high setting for 30 seconds. Blend with the mixer again until smooth.
- ➢ Empty into the prepared pan (1-inch layer). Cover & chill for two hours in the fridge.
- ➢ Slice into 12 portions.
- ➢ Serve and enjoy or store in the fridge for a delicious treat later.

NUTRITION INFORMATION: Calories: 242 Carbs: 4.4 g Protein: 2.6 g Fat: 25.3 g

Thank you for reading this book

CPSIA information can be obtained
at www.ICGtesting.com
Printed in the USA
BVHW061112030521
606339BV00004B/521

9 781802 670899